Reviews

Helen Johnson has not rushed into print. She has taken a lifetime to develop and refine a therapy for diagnosing and treating trauma and twenty-five years to write about it. Starting with her own personal journey, in the face of many challenges, she courageously pressed on to arrive at an understanding of her condition and a means of treating it. Now, her insights have released a passion to let the world know. In essence, Helen's book is a teaching aid and tool to help those who are interested in understanding the after effects of shock and trauma, and should bring relief to many sufferers.

— Noel Braun, author of *I Guess I'll Keep on Walking*

Experienced author, Helen Johnson's *Trauma Free – Your Five Steps to Freedom*, comes onto the Australian book market at precisely the right time. The present moment in 2020, needs a book to address PTSD. (Post Traumatic Stress disorder)

Helen is quick to point out in the outset of the book that the levels of severity of Trauma vary significantly from family to family and person to person. She also sheds light that there are biological and chemical changes in the body. Recounting her own journey through PTSD, she shows she has a mission in life to help others. To quote Helen, "Adrenalin is the right response for fight or flight, but not for everyday living."

In Helen's own time of need, she found help woefully wanting. Her light bulb moment was when she "decided to let go of some of my emotional pain, stop feeling sorry for myself and start taking responsibility for my own life."

I found the following the most useful tool — In order to come through PTSD, the horrific pictures in our heads have to be found, confronted and defeated.

Thank you Helen for sharing your story and showing all those who have suffered traumatic episodes in their lives, a way through the pain to a Trauma Free future.

— Judith Flitcroft, author of *Walk Back in Time*

Written with such honesty and clarity, offering hope and guidance dealing with long-term trauma.

An emotional, must read personal journey, bound to resonate with many.

— Vivian Waring, author of *When Tears Ran Dry*

TRAUMA FREE

Your Five Steps to Freedom

'Helen's personal story is ... courageous!'
— **John Bugge**

Helen Elizabeth Johnson

Published in Australia by Sid Harta Publishers Pty Ltd,
ABN: 46 119 415 842
23 Stirling Crescent, Glen Waverley, Victoria 3150 Australia
Telephone: +61 3 9560 9920, Facsimile: +61 3 9545 1742
E-mail: author@sidharta.com.au

Helen Johnson Australia
Email: helenjohnsonhealth508@gmail.com

©Copyright: 2019 Helen Elizabeth Johnson. All rights reserved. No part of this publication may be reproduced, stored in a retrieval system or transmitted in any form by any means without the prior permission of the copyright owner.

Inquiries should be made to the publisher.

Every effort has been made to ensure that this book is free from error or omissions. However, the Publisher, the Author, the Editor or their respective employees or agents, shall not accept responsibility for injury, loss or damage occasioned to any person acting or refraining from action because of the material in this book, whether or not such injury, loss or damage is in any way due to any negligent act or omission, breach of duty or default on the part of the Publisher, the Author, the Editor, or their respective employees or agents.

Author: Helen Elizabeth Johnson
ISBN: 978-1-925707-09-0

Title: **TRAUMA FREE. Your Five Steps to Freedom.**

Subjects: Pain, flashbacks — pictures, anger, fear, loneliness, abandonment, suicide, depression, anxiety, headaches, exhaustion, mood swings, the mind never stops chattering, nervous tension, always feeling restless or the opposite never wanting to do anything, etc.

If *you* are interested in understanding and healing trauma, this story of healing personal and generational trauma is for you.

Australia Editor: Barbara Ivusic, Sydney/Germany

Cover: Colleen Keith Design

ALSO PUBLISHED BY HELEN JOHNSON

"Natural Stress and Anxiety Relief."
How to Use the Johnson Breathing Technique.
The Adrenaline Connection. Published 2008.

Available in libraries in Australia
and from www.amazon.com

CONTENTS

Dedication		ix
Testimonial — John Bugge		xi
Introduction		1
Part I	Post-Traumatic Stress Disorder	5
Part II	'Trauma Therapy'	73
Part III	'Trauma Therapy'- **Five Steps** —shortened version	121
Part IV	2017 Trauma Free update	125
Part V	An Overview and Conclusion 2020	127

I dedicate this book to my father.

TESTIMONIAL

Helen Johnson's publication, *Trauma Free*, is a clear and compassionate study of the stress and trauma that can be brought into the family home. I was an Australian Army conscript in Vietnam and I can fully understand and identify with her family's story. When I returned home, I did not realise the degree of my guilt which remained hidden and untreated, but after four decades it surfaced with Australia's invasion of Iraq in 2003.

Helen's personal story is fascinating and courageous, and I especially commend the section on 'Trauma Therapy' which provides an uncomplicated explanation for diagnosing and treating trauma.

John Bugge
Portarlington
Australia
April 2017

INTRODUCTION

The term Post-Traumatic Stress Disorder (PTSD) first appeared in 1980 in the third edition of the Diagnostic and Statistical Manual of Mental Disorders (DSM-lll) published by the American Psychiatric Association. It was used to describe a disorder returning Vietnam veterans were experiencing, caused by their involvement on the battlefield of war.

One of the earliest records of war related PTSD could have been made by the Greek historian Herodotus in 490BCE when he wrote about the emotional strain associated with war. He described how, during the Battle of Marathon, an Athenian soldier who suffered no injury became blind after witnessing the death of a fellow soldier.

Over the last few centuries various names have been given to disorders showing symptoms similar to PTSD. These include Nostalgia and Homesickness - Wars in Europe throughout the 17th and 18th Centuries; Soldier Heart – the American Civil War, 19th Century; Shell Shock – WWI, Battle

Fatigue – WWII, Post-Traumatic Stress Disorder (PTSD) – Vietnam, all in the 20th Century.

PTSD is a mental disorder that recognises how short and long term trauma, the after effect of shock, affects people's lives. This isn't limited to ones work and home life, but can also affect their health and wellbeing.

Today other terms and phrases have been added to the never-ending list recognizing the various effects of shock resulting in Trauma, these include - Human Devastation Syndrome (HDS), and Complex-Post-Traumatic Stress Disorder (C-PTSD). The phrase HDS came about because of the appalling atrocities associated with the war in Syria and C-PTSD focuses on and describes, among other symptoms the emotions and feelings associated with long-term and/or chronic PTSD.

As a result of the work and research I have undertaken I have coined a new phrase, **Post Emotional Shock/Trauma (PEST)**, which separates emotional illness from mental illness.

PTSD and **PEST** both cause biological and chemical changes in the body and mind, however I believe many professionals in both the non-medical and the medical fields link PTSD to mental illness with little regard to it being possibly an emotional illness. I too was focused there until I had the sudden realisation that I needed to intellectually separate emotional illness from mental illness.

Changing my diagnostic focus from PTSD to using the principals of **Post Emotional Shock/Trauma (PEST)** and the five steps of **'Trauma Therapy'** has brought about miraculous results and is the reason why this book which has taken me decades to write, is now finished.

The story I am telling here is my story. Firstly, it is about how generational PTSD affected my extended family after my father returned from World War II suffering Anxiety Neurosis (PTSD). Secondly, it explains in detail how the generational PTSD symptoms I experienced early in life compounded whenever I found myself later in life in threatening or frightening situations. Thirdly, it describes how 'Trauma Therapy' evolved and fourthly, it describes the amazing relief I felt when I finally found the answers I was looking for.

***Trauma Free*, Your Five Steps to Freedom** has helped me improve my mental, physical and emotional health and well-being, bringing greater joy, peace, happiness and freedom into my life.

It worked for me, it can work for you!

Please Note: Dyslexia and shock and trauma had equal effect on my life and even though I can understand how debilitating Dyslexia can be, I decided when writing this book — *Trauma*

Free, Your Five Steps to Freedom, to concentrate on what I could change e.g. the effect of shock and trauma on my life, rather than on what I could not change — Dyslexia.

PART I
Post-Traumatic Stress Disorder

This book -*Trauma Free, Your Five Steps to Freedom* — is about parallel lives. It tells the life stories of two completely different people both of whom suffered a mental illness Post/Traumatic Stress Disorder, (PTSD).

The first story is my father's story; he was a World War II veteran. The second story is my own story, the life story of an ordinary civilian. The conclusion reached, however, after decades of research is far from ordinary. It is extra-ordinary!

The programming was there right from the beginning!

As my father stood looking proudly at his first born, one-hour old baby girl, the Sister-in-Charge of the maternity ward leaned forward and whispered: 'Matron said, she is the ugliest baby ever born in this hospital!'

What a shock!

I wonder what my father thought and felt on hearing those ominous words spoken about me, his beautiful newborn little girl.

To this day I do not know what my father thought, or what he felt when he heard those words. I do know, however, that unfortunately he went straight away from there to tell my mother what had been said and my mother was to unkindly remind me of those words many times in the following years. The ripple effect of those harsh, damaging words somehow affected me personally on a profound level for most of my life.

AN UGLY LIFE

I was born into a fear-filled environment in 1940 under the umbrella of potential Post-Traumatic Stress Disorder.

World War II was in full swing and because Australia was so far from the war zone on the other side of the world, life for me, the newborn, we thought would go on as usual when the war ended. But that was not to be.

War changed everything!

Without warning my life and the lives of our family members were changed forever when my father came home from WWII in 1945. He was discharged with medically diagnosed anxiety and a stress disorder — shell shock. Shell shock, years later was renamed Post-Traumatic Stress Disorder (PTSD).

My PTSD story began in those early years and it was only when thinking about my life when writing this book that I understood just how subtly insidious and destructive to a person's healthy development that life lived with generational and/or personal PTSD could be.

In my early years, world leaders were in control. They held the umbrella of fear and potential PTSD over our heads as we wondered what the outcome of World War II would be.

Within five years the outcome was clear and it was not long before the generational damage to humanity from PTSD was being recognised, first by the individuals who were affected by the symptoms of the disorder personally and, secondly, by the families who were forced to live with the changed personalities of those affected individuals.

PTSD is about shock and trauma!

Trauma follows shock. Trauma is the mental, physical and emotional condition that affects both mind and body following a shock.

Physically, shock causes the nervous system, the engine that drives the body to automatically enter its survival mode. Survival mode alters the body's breathing pattern as it activates the body's *fight or flight* response. The *fight or flight* response then causes the body to start running on adrenaline.

When the moment of shock has passed, the body should be allowed to return to normal, i.e., the nervous system should be given time to settle down so that the body stops running on adrenaline.

If the body does not return to normal, the symptoms associated with PTSD may appear and escalate out of control. Over time these symptoms may also become permanent causing a person to suffer high levels of distress, anxiety and sickness, mentally, physically and emotionally. Trauma is a person's mental, physical and emotional response to an emotional shock. Animals deal with shock much more efficiently than humans!

If an animal suffers a shock and is frightened its body responds in a similar way to the human body. In fear, most animals go into hiding, running as far away as they can from everyone and everything until the effect of the shock subsides, and the nervous system settles down.

Withdrawing in this way helps to stop most animals being traumatised permanently.

Human beings, however, do not run away and hide when frightened, they keep going and unfortunately do not take the time to recognise that the whole body, (mind and body), has suffered a shock and is therefore traumatised. Not running away leaves the human body susceptible to being permanently traumatised.

To authenticate the credibility of 'Trauma Therapy,' the therapy I developed to help myself heal from the devastating effect of generational and personal PTSD, I need to go back to 1948 and my sister's **brush with death.** This was a terrifying experience for me because I was blamed for letting it happen.

Our family was holidaying miles from a town on my uncle's farm in North Western Victoria, Australia, and there was no doctor close by.

We children: my cousin, my sister and my brother were annoying our mothers who wanted to have a quiet chat before dinner. My mother turned to us saying, 'go outside and play for a while,' and looking straight at me, she added, 'don't let your sister go near the hay.'

Being two years younger than me and the owner of a very strong, stubborn, determined nature, the first thing my sister did when we went outside was run straight into the hay.

Immediately she started coughing, coughing, and coughing!

At the time, I didn't know if she was having an asthma attack or if she just had a piece of hay stuck in her throat. I thought it was asthma because she had suffered from asthma attacks before, except that this time she could not catch her breath or stop coughing and I began to feel very scared.

I immediately started screaming and yelled for Mum to come and help me. She rushed out and took my sister inside with her. I can clearly remember the sequence of events because when Mum took my sister inside, she left me standing where she had found us, and I didn't know what to do next. I didn't know whether I should follow them inside or stay where I was.

That night no one wanted to talk to me or listen to me, they were all furious with me. I tried verbally to defend myself, but no one wanted to hear me. They ignored me, turned their backs and walked away from me when I tried to explain what had happened. I was devastated. I wanted them to hear that it was not all my fault. Tears were running down my cheeks as I silently sobbed. I wanted them to listen, but they ignored me. I wanted them to know that my sister went into the hay behind my back when I was checking to see where our cousin was. My cousin was only four, four years younger than me, and I was concerned for her safety, I wanted to know if she had come out to play with us. She hadn't.

I was frightened for my sister and felt both shocked and upset by what was happening to her. But, due to my young age and not really understanding the severity of the situation, or what the outcome might be, I had no clue that she could die! She had had many asthma attacks before and I was upset more for me than anyone else because no one would listen to me. I can remember feeling utterly helpless and powerless as I was ignored when unbeknown to me an innocent event nearly became a major tragedy.

I was shaking all over and felt sick to my stomach. To this day, I can still remember how useless and helpless I felt standing there in the kitchen with tears running down my face, my head hanging down in shame and my arms dangling uselessly by my sides. Even though I was quite tall for my age, I felt tiny standing there wondering if anyone would ever believe me or trust me again.

As my energy drained away, all sorts of emotions started flooding through me. I felt confused, frightened, lost, alone, and very guilty because even though I knew that I should accept some of the blame and wanted to, I also knew that my sister was partly to blame for what happened. But no one would talk to me. I lay in bed fully awake through that long night. I can remember thinking as I lay there that, other than the sound of my sister's coughing and raspy breathing, just how still, dark and quiet everything was both inside and outside the farmhouse as we all waited to see what would happen.

My punishment was severe! I was sent to bed without dinner and left alone for the rest of the night. I was really frightened and hungry and didn't have a clue about what was happening. I lay on the bed for hours, rigid with fear, listening to my own panic breathing. My heartbeat sounded like thunder in my ears. I was in shock myself, panicking, terribly short of breath and became more so as the night dragged on.

Personally, I was worried about people not liking me, and it took me quite a while to awaken to the fact that it was not about me but about the survival of my sister.

With the innocence of childhood, my concern was for only me. I could not understand why everyone seemed to hate me; I couldn't figure out why they were ignoring me and didn't want to talk to me.

Suddenly, my sister's coughing stopped. In fear, I curled up into the foetal position for what was left of the night and waited for someone to come and tell me whether my sister was dead or alive. But no one came!

I felt real terror that night and realised later in life, as I clutched my own personal PTSD umbrella close to my heart that life wasn't as simple as I had thought, the shock of my sister's brush with death and the behaviour of others towards me changed my way of looking at life forever!

I started growing up that night!

The next morning when I crept out of bed to go to breakfast, I was greeted by the sight of my sister, happily the centre of attention, sitting eating breakfast as if nothing had happened.

She was suffering no ill effects from her night of drama. She had pulled through as she had done many times before.

Nothing had changed!

Obviously, everyone was happy for her; but something had changed! I felt different and sensed a shift in everyone's attitude towards me as I was still being ignored. This time something had really changed. I sat there at the table feeling sad and lonely. I felt guilty and ashamed like an outsider, as if I was the cause of everything that had happened the night before. My shoulders slumped, and my head dropped forward as I wondered if I would ever be included in any future family conversations.

At that young age, I didn't understand that I was in *shock* and it was years before I became aware of how badly I was traumatised by that shock. It was also years before I could learn not to feel fear every time my sister had an asthma attack.

By the time I was ten, I was experiencing severe trauma, and my fortyyearold father was chronically traumatised. Both of us, suffering different levels of PTSD!

My father's PTSD was already recognised. My own PTSD, however, went unrecognised for years until I started asking myself questions about why my life was so different from everyone else's, and it was many more years before I had the courage to stop hiding and face the outside world so that I could start answering some of those questions.

Up to the age of ten, I was relatively healthy, and my behaviour patterns were, as far as I knew, typical for my age. However, from then on, and through my teenage years, some unusual behaviours and mood swings surfaced. This made things more difficult for me at home and I could not understand the emotional distance that was growing between me and my family, I felt totally isolated from them and very lonely. At the time I hid those feelings, but they got worse as the years passed by.

What I just wanted was my family's love and approval. I know now, that when I did not get what I wanted, I converted what should have been anger at their bad attitudes and behaviours towards me into suppressed feelings of hurt and defeat. It took me many years using 'Trauma Therapy' to uncover those pains, mainly because I did not know what was missing. It was years before I realised that it was a lack of love and approval from within my family that was missing.

MY FATHER'S STORY

I do not have any substantial information about my father's younger years. But as far as I know, before joining the Navy and suffering anxiety and PTSD, my father was a normal, healthy, fully employed, active person who loved sports, especially sailing and football.

After enlisting in the Navy he had a distinguished career as, first, a cadet in early 1942 then rising to Captain of his ship, Nepean by the end of that year. Unfortunately by then he had lost a man overboard and silently blamed himself for the loss until he died in his seventies.

At his funeral, a representative from Legacy showed me a file, (these files are now sealed so I cannot confirm that this information is correct), with Dad's war history in it. He said that Dad had lived 'parallel lives', (the term he used). The life we saw him living on the outside, and a life he lived within himself on the inside — one of fear. Fear of being court-marshalled from losing a man overboard.

When I told my mother about the file, she answered me saying, 'I wrote to your father every day during the war to make sure he didn't commit suicide. He was always threatening with that.' When I further questioned her, she would not tell me anything else, and I can clearly remember Mum sitting at the desk in our lounge room writing her daily letters.

The shock of losing a man overboard, and the ensuing symptoms of trauma which are associated with PTSD, severely impacted the rest of my father's life, my life, and indirectly the lives of all our family members.

For his whole working life, after the end of the war, my father robotically, went to work at eight o'clock in the morning and returned home at six o'clock in the evening when he withdrew into a world of his own. It seemed to me that he never spoke to me or anyone else.

We lived in a culture of silence. My mother was always saying, 'don't make a noise, don't upset your father,' and because she had always wanted to be a nurse, she now focused her attention on nursing both my sister with her asthma and my dad with his PTSD as they continued being ill.

Then, happy days for my mother, after the war ended, my brother was born!

Many years later I was still searching for answers as to why my life didn't seem to be the same as other peoples. One day in desperation I rang my mother's best friend. She was in her nineties by then and very alert. I asked her straight out, 'what was really wrong in our family?' She answered immediately, 'Your mother only ever loved one person, your brother.'

As soon as I heard her answer I knew she was right. Instantly, I understood why I was always ignored and left feeling abandoned and unimportant. I was a female, not a male! I may have been their first born, an important position I thought, but I was never to be the healthy son and heir who would carry the family name into the future as my brother was expected to do, and to make matters worse, I was never sick. It was true, Mum had only two loves in her life that she lived for — my brother and nursing. This meant that she didn't have time to pay attention to anyone or anything else. Not a social life, not her beautiful singing voice, not me, or my sister unless she was sick; and not my father.

How sad! In different ways, we all missed out on our mother's love, and in retrospect, I also wondered how much my mother's own personal dreams may have faded with each succeeding year? PTSD really did affect us all, often in unrecognised ways.

I was nearly five-years-old when the war ended, and I can clearly remember the happiness everyone on our street shared with one another as we celebrated.

My family's happiness, however, totally reversed when Dad arrived home. He was discharged as medically unfit from the Navy. He came back under the shadow of suicide; the happiness we had all shared the day the war ended quickly dispersed. For our family, that happiness was gone forever!

Much has been written about medically diagnosed PTSD and I do not wish to comment on that here. Simply stated, having suffered and triumphed over PTSD myself, I wish I had rebelled a little less, behaved a little better and offered my mother and father more understanding and love. Apparently, they must have gone through a great deal themselves in those years … in hindsight I know I did not make their lives any easier.

I now understand some of the reasons for this lack of understanding and rather than write about medically diagnosed PTSD, I would like to share more of my own story with you. It may act as a guide, and help you understand trauma.

GENERATIONAL PTSD

I was not a sickly child and did not need nursing during my early years. Thus, I didn't get any special love and attention which every child needs and deserves. I didn't get the love, attention and mentoring that I needed, except from the Christian teachings I received from going to Sunday school and church every Sunday.

Church and Sunday school taught me to forgive and love everyone, no matter what happened. Those teachings taught me to turn the other cheek, (turn away, walk away and forgive them), love others even when things go wrong. I heard inspiring words every Sunday telling me everyone should love me as I loved them, but my home-life demonstrated the opposite.

I was receiving confused and disjointed subliminal messages, which I found hard to interpret at home, at school and at church and I did not always know how to think or behave at home, school or church. Everything I did seemed to bring the wrong results for me mainly, I now know, because I was pleasing others, especially my mother, instead of myself! This pattern of forgiving, no matter what, taught me to be powerless to meet my own needs and it was decades before I learned to stand up for myself and fight to get my own needs met.

As I grew up, outside in the real world I was successful and well-liked. I was given lots of positions of responsibility and authority in my pre-teen and teen years. These included: class captain, school captain, leading roles in Girl Guides, tennis team captain, etc. None of these honours, however, gave me any real enjoyment because I had neither support, nor approval coming from within my home and no approval or rewards for good works. Home was, for me, stressful! I always felt anxious and nervous from trying to help others get their needs met. It was all about pleasing them as best I could just to keep the peace so that I wouldn't get into trouble.

One example of what my home life was like occurred when I was awarded the honour of being named head prefect of the private girls' school I attended. Ours was a small class, and even though I had given some thought as to who might be named head prefect, it did not occur to me that I might be chosen.

During a school assembly near the end of my second last year at the school the Headmistress stood up to make an announcement. Everyone became very quiet and attentive and into the silence she said, our head prefect for next year will be Helen Johnson. I was totally shocked and just stood there stunned as everyone started clapping, patting me on the back and wishing me well.

I felt both proud and excited and could not wait to go home and share my good news with Mum. However, as the time to leave school came closer I had a bad feeling about returning home and started delaying my arrival time, arriving about an hour and a half after my sister.

Fearing that there could be something wrong with my achievement, I went straight to my bedroom through the back door to give myself time to pluck up the courage to tell Mum my good news.

Eventually, I walked into the kitchen where my mother and sister were talking. I waited for a lull in their conversation and said, 'I was made head prefect today, for next year.' My mother half-turned to me and said, 'I know, I'll have to buy a new hat because the service is in the Church of England, not in our own church.'

Then, she turned her back on me and went on with the conversation she was having with my sister. I felt so disappointed, defeated and angry, and I can remember thinking I was right to be scared to tell Mum of my achievement. The little self-confidence I had flowed out of me; deep down I had hoped that Mum would be proud of me and approve of my success. But, none of that was forthcoming. I desperately wanted and needed Mum and Dad's approval, and I felt terribly hurt and deeply disappointed when I didn't get any acknowledgement at all.

How was I to deal with being ignored, how was I to change this situation, I asked myself?

When Mum turned away from me without congratulating me or giving me a hug, I had an instant thought, of course, my sister arriving home before me had already given Mum the news. At that moment I felt totally betrayed, this had been the most exciting day of my life and no-one cared or was one bit interested.

To add insult to injury, my father said nothing.

TEENAGE YEARS — A DIFFICULT HOME LIFE

Suddenly I knew that 'growing up' would make no difference. I knew that nothing I could ever do or be would be good enough to win approval from my family or make them change their attitudes towards me.

Now I asked myself again, how was I going to deal with the anger that was building up in me?

Even though I felt as though I would blow up with the anger I was feeling I kept it hidden inside me until I went to bed at night. In bed I cried it out of me into my pillow. Each morning I would remember what I had been taught in church and I did my best to forgive them, love them and let go of my pain.

Most of the time I felt like two different people, and I am sure I behaved like two different people. Every day I felt more confused with the mixed messages I was giving myself and getting from others. I always felt different and somehow disconnected from everyone and everything and often asked myself what was wrong with me, was this me doing this to me, or, was my family doing this to me. Mostly I blamed myself and thought I could put everything right on my own but it took years of attending many different self-help courses before I could change anything. All the courses helped in some way but it was 'Trauma Therapy', the therapy I developed myself that finally freed me from my confusing and traumatic past.

I was really hurting and started consciously keeping my distance from others. This somehow separated me even further from my family.

There were no mentors or anyone else to ask advice of in those days as there is today and gradually, as I moved into my teens and the swinging fifties, the pendulum of my own withdrawal and isolation from everyone swung the other way as I found boys and an exciting adrenaline-driven social world, away from home.

I did what many other teenagers were doing I broke out with the wrong sort of behaviour and bounced from one bad and often shocking decision and activity to another.

There was, however, an upside or two to my feelings of being unable to communicate easily with adults. In my mid-teen years, we had a pervert living across from us; it used to amaze me how often he was standing in our driveway, partly hidden by the shadow of the fence and the trees in the garden next door. He was always there when Mum, Dad, and the rest of my family were not home. The whole situation scared me, but I couldn't tell my parents that he was there almost daily, because I was sure they would not believe me.

Years later, I understood that although I tended to talk too much and too loudly at times to get attention and fill the silences at home, I found that I was unable to easily communicate with adult strangers. I realised that because I did not get enough practice talking to adults at home. I became tongue-tied when it came to general conversations with them. Thus, I did not have the necessary skills to carry on a conversation with this man. He was an adult, and because adults rarely communicated with me, lucky for me, he and I could not communicate easily.

There were also three personal reasons why I couldn't communicate easily with this man. First, I was timid and conservative and somehow knew that what he was saying to me and showing me, was wrong. Being shy, I felt really embarrassed looking at the playing card-size pictures of what today would be called sexy women most of them wearing few or no clothes.

My second reason was that I was scared the neighbours might see me talking to him, tell Mum and Dad, and I would be in big trouble for flirting; and third, I hated the thought of accepting the invitations he was always giving me to go swimming in his pool.

I had heard the neighbours gossiping about 'the shame of his family and visitors swimming in his pool with no clothes on.' These were the fifties and even though times were changing I knew I didn't want to break society's rules; I knew I definitely did not want to go swimming in his pool without wearing a swimsuit.

There was another time, however, when during my secondary school years that limited communication, conversational skills and lack of understanding of the English language positively affected me.

Studying the English language and learning the plays of William Shakespeare had always been a huge problem for me because I had difficulty understanding the sophisticated Shakespearian language.

One day, our English Literature teacher called me aside after school, stood over me and said, 'I can see that you 'hate' Shakespeare. But, if you want to pass the exam, I suggest you learn the work by heart.'

'Then, after that, you can 'choose' to read whatever you want to read.' She then turned, and with her head held high, marched away from me without a backward glance.

I stood there for a while thinking about what she had said; I decided to obey her. I learned as much as I could by heart and passed the exam with flying colours. Before that time, because I was so busy 'trying' to be part of my family I had never taken the time to read many books. From then on, I became more mindful of my own needs and started reading everything in sight. This was a real plus for me, and I thank her to this day for challenging me. I have never lost my love of books and reading.

Reading took my mind off what was happening at home and helped me fill my knowledge vacuum. I still had trouble conversing with adults, but I was able gradually to broaden my educational horizons. A great gift indeed!

Reading was the only time in my life when my mother's words concerning Dad, 'Don't upset your father,' (meaning don't make a noise, or talk too much), really worked. If I read a book I was quiet — this pleased everyone!

The poor communication skills I had, meant the pervert had a hard time starting up a conversation with me. That gave me the time I needed to escape to the safety of my family house, and my teacher gave me the greatest of gifts, she opened my world up to books, and the joy of reading. She offered me a new reality in the freedom of choice. She also gave me a sense of release from the pressures I was living under. I could now change my behaviour, choose to read a book instead of worrying about the things I could not change.

Being locked out of practising verbal communication with adults at home has been detrimental to me all my life as far as social networking is concerned. Lack of verbal practice in those early years and unfortunately, even today, caused me to make some very embarrassing verbal gaffes (spoken statements) socially, especially when I relax and am part of a friendly social group.

I seem to let my guard down and forget to think about what I am saying, just like I did under pressure at home when I was trying to connect. At home, I was ignored or was told to be quiet but I did not have that boundary offered to me socially and sometimes kept going when I should have stopped talking. Very embarrassing!

Today, — there is a stunned silence as I try to cover my gaffe, but it never works, I end up being ignored, looked at in a funny way by others and feel guilty myself for causing a break in the flow of the conversation. If situations like this continue to happen one tends to lose one's self-esteem and desire to mix socially and that awful feeling of loneliness takes over again.

My teenage years were confusing for me. Now, I was attracting the wrong sort of attention from both my family at home and from outsiders. Once again, in the middle of all this, I was brought back down to earth by my mother when she reminded me of my ugliness.

Boys had come into my life, and I was attempting to make myself more attractive for one boy in particular, he was going to the same dance I was going to, at our local church. I was sitting at the kitchen table asking for Mum's help while I tried to put my thick, straight, strong, blonde hair into curlers. Suddenly, Mum turned to me and reminded me of the nasty comment the Sister in the hospital had made about me the day I was born.

Defeated, I picked up my things and went to my room. I was really shocked at being reminded of the words the Sister in the hospital had said to my father when I was born and I was even more shocked to hear my mother repeat those words to me again especially when I was trying to make myself more beautiful.

My self-esteem was already at its lowest because of teenage skin and hormonal problems and hearing those words once again touched me in a place buried deep inside me. The little self-esteem I had built up over time disappeared that day. And, all for nothing! To compound the pain, the boy did not turn up at the dance.

THE IN BETWEEN YEARS — AWAY FROM HOME

As I mentioned earlier, even though I lacked self-confidence and struggled with my lack of communication skills outside of the home, I was in both the business and social worlds fairly successful. I made friends easily and quickly rose to positions of authority that carried great responsibility at work.

Happily, in my early twenties, I married; but, it lasted for only a short time. I think my lack of suitable role models in my growing up years and lack of adequate communication skills were the primary causes of the marital breakup. As always I blamed myself and a very miserable time followed as I successfully opened my protective, wounded person PTSD umbrella to look after myself. Withdrawal was all I knew! It was the only way I knew that could help me hide from everyone as I sadly went through my three long years of waiting for the divorce to be finalised.

Withdrawing into myself, I started learning what it felt like to face life completely alone. Lack of understanding, loneliness, and abandonment are three of the biggest issues for anyone suffering PTSD and I was no different.

I was utterly traumatised and missed the habitual comfort of thinking I had a caring family. I was no longer welcome at home. I was in my mid-twenties and this time they really weren't there for me! Those years were some of the hardest and loneliest years of my life. Being a 'divorced woman,' I was a total disgrace in the eyes of both my childhood authorities — my family and my church.

I had nowhere to go and I felt terribly ashamed of my situation. I knew I was an embarrassment to my family and most of my friends, and the rift that was already there between family, the few friends who were left and the church further widened. I felt as though I wasn't wanted by anyone because especially my family made little effort to contact me. I knew I was never to be forgiven for getting a divorce, and that really hurt. Marriage was forever, I had broken one of the cardinal rules of life at that time. Married people did not divorce!

As I peered out of the window of the single room I rented in a boarding house near where I worked, my future looked bleak. Added to all the other problems I had, I now had to learn to live through the disgrace of being a divorcee.

The highs and lows of life were beginning to take their toll. I was exhausted from running on the adrenaline of fear, wearing a mask, and pretending there was nothing wrong. I was still trying to please everyone to avoid adding more feelings of hurt and guilt to how I already felt if I did something wrong and got the blame.

I loved the adrenaline rush and the fuss that was made when I did well, but after the highs always followed the lows and with them came depression.

Depression for me was a big black empty space, a hole which I felt that I would never climb out of.

Sometimes I stayed depressed for months, while always wearing a mask of happiness so others could not see what was happening within me. My reasoning was, I didn't know what was going on with me and didn't know what was wrong either, so how could I expect anyone else to know what was wrong with me or help me if I couldn't explain my problems.

Like my father, I did think about suicide. But, I never imagined ways to accomplish it. Years later, I realised I only thought about suicide but deep down knew that I didn't want to die anyway. What I wanted was answers!

Within me, I had a driving force that really wanted to live and know what was wrong with my thinking. I wanted to know why I felt that I was different from other people, and why my family treated me differently.

I asked myself, 'why have I always yearned for answers'? I wanted to know how I could improve my life but, how?

Some PTSD sufferers stay in the same place for years and never move. But, the opposite — moving, is also one of the restless characteristics associated with PTSD. For me, I needed to keep moving; it kept my adrenaline flowing. That, in turn, kept me moving. Without knowing it, I was caught in an unbreakable loop.

I was looking for answers and thought I would find them in the next course I did or in the next place I moved to.

Eventually, I did recognise that the answers were within me, but that time was a long way off in those years.

Living with nervous tension and stress caused me to feel really exhausted. I wondered if I was suffering from Chronic Fatigue Syndrome because I always seemed to be too tired to think straight, often making dubious, hasty, sometimes rash decisions that were not properly thought through. Yes, decisions that made me more vulnerable to being impacted by the adverse effects of further mistakes including various levels of shock that occurred whenever I moved.

Still, I used to think arrogantly, I did quite well handling all those adjustments, that is, until 1970!

ADULT YEARS AND MY OWN PERSONAL PTSD

In 1970, twenty odd years after my sister's brush with death, everything changed for me forever. It was in this year that I was to suffer my own near-death experience.

I was twenty-nine, married, with a stepdaughter, and a five-month old son of our own. We lived on a small farm quite some miles from a tiny town, in a well-known country area, in southern Australia.

The one hundred and twenty-year-old red brick, farmhouse we lived in, was situated on a slight rise well back from a remote country road. This particular night I can remember thinking as I looked out of the window at the surrounding countryside, just how peaceful and quiet the evening was. Our children were in bed, and I was feeling happy, relaxed and satisfied with myself after a long and busy, but fulfilling day.

The day's events included talking to my father on the telephone. My mother had suffered a stroke, and my dad said she was feeling a little better. This was good news. Our nearest neighbours, who lived a few miles away, had visited us during the day and kindly offered to give us help or advice on any farming matters we may need assistance with. We were new to farming, and I can remember thinking what wonderful, friendly people country people are.

They, however, were unable to be of any assistance to me with what happened over the next few hours. What happened came out of nowhere!

That evening, while I was brushing my hair in preparation for going to bed, someone jumped me, attacking me from behind. Suddenly I felt strong hands squeezing my throat and neck. I was forced off the stool I was sitting on down to the floor. I knew I was being strangled, but I could not react due to the strength of the person overpowering me. I fought to get my breath and gasped for air as I fell to the floor.

I can remember hitting the back of my head very hard on the edge of the stool I had been sitting on as I went down. I started to let go within myself sensing that I was going to lose consciousness, and can remember feeling the weirdest feeling creeping over me, all through my body.

As the blackness of shock overtook me, I lost all ability to think for myself. I was quickly losing control and was unable to consciously think or act rationally.

My mind was still working at some level registering what was happening, but I was unable to command my body to do anything. Having no control stopped me from thinking. I could not think what I needed to do to help myself. It stopped me from thinking about what action message I should send to my body to tell it what to do to help me. I felt so strange, and lost all perception of time. I couldn't tell whether I was on the floor for two minutes or two hours.

Sometime later, I started thinking in a detached way about what to do to help myself. I could see that I had not fallen flat on the floor, but I was in some sort of misshapen sitting position leaning on my right arm and hand. Shortly I become aware of the pain I could feel, in the back of my head and neck; it was excruciating and I also felt a throbbing pain in the back of my head. This pain started to overpower me, and once again I couldn't think straight. I couldn't think what to do. I didn't know what I needed to do to stop the pain. I couldn't decide whether to let myself fall flat down onto the floor or stay where I was, half sitting and half lying down.

I must have lost consciousness; because when I woke up, I found that I had fallen over and was lying, face down flat on the floor. Lying there, I realised, as I started to regain consciousness that I was now paralysed. I couldn't move, and I couldn't see or know where the person who had done this to me was.

I had never felt so scared, or so much fear and terror in my life!

I didn't know it at the time, but I was in shock and so physically, mentally and emotionally traumatised by this second major shock in my life that I could not move. I couldn't get up off the floor without falling over.

I felt so disoriented and disconnected from myself that when I did begin to think about moving, I found I couldn't remember how to move or walk. I had no idea where the door to the bedroom was, and couldn't escape even if I wanted to. Now I felt really terrified! I felt totally disconnected from my normal self, and my thinking faculties seemed to have left me. I felt as though there was an empty space deep in the middle of my head where my brain should have been.

Gradually my automatic adrenaline-driven personal survival system activated itself and I slowly sat up, then carefully leaning over onto my hands and knees I started to crawl.

At first, I had no feeling in my hands and knees and crawling was difficult, but my main difficulty was remembering how to crawl when I was very unsteady and shaking like a leaf. Gradually, I began to feel a sense of relief as the feeling came back into my hands and knees and I managed to get up off the floor and started stumbling towards where I thought the door was. My feet felt as though they did not belong to me because they did not seem to know what they should do or where they should go. I felt like a baby, a newborn, who didn't have a clue about how to walk.

As my thinking cleared, I started to regain some sense of balance. I don't know how long it took me, but eventually, I found the door to the bedroom and wandered down the hallway. I swerved from one side of the hall to the other on my way to the kitchen. All I could think of in those moments was that I wanted a cup of tea!

When looking back over the past and specifically at that night, I realised that learning to walk was just the beginning. Those steps, I took then, were literally the first steps I took into a new life. They were the steps I needed to take metaphorically as I started to *learn* how to do *everything* from scratch as I learned how to live again. I discovered that, nothing I had known previously came naturally anymore!

Making a cup of tea should have been a simple routine. I had made many cups of tea in the past. To this day I cannot remember what I did the night of the attack, but early the next morning making a cup of tea was a new experience for me.

When I went into the kitchen that next morning I automatically switched the kitchen lights on and flicked the switch to start the jug boiling, these were typically routine actions. However, as I watched my hands put the tea into the pot and reach for the jug to pour the boiled water onto the tea leaves and then pour the brewed tea into the cup I saw the strangest thing. I could *see* that one hand was holding the teapot and the other hand the teacup and I could *see* that the hand holding the cup and the arm it was connected to was physically connected to my shoulder but, it did not *feel* as though there was a connection. There was no feeling between the top of my arm and my body. This really did frighten me, and once again I started to feel as though I was passing out.

I thought to myself, oh no, not again! The shock of seeing one thing and feeling another caused that weird feeling to start engulfing me again. This time I fought the feeling and stayed upright and in control. I knew I was still somehow separated but was able to continue watching as if from a distance what was happening to me. I understood many years later that the conscious and subconscious parts of my brain were having great difficulty knowing how to get me working.

I knew that my fingers could feel the china of the cup, but there seemed to be no feeling of connection between the arm and me. Also, there was darkness between my arm, the arm holding the cup and my body and I can remember thinking how dark everything was, even though I knew I had switched the kitchen lights on.

I don't know how long this went on, but because I was conditioned over many years not to ask for help when I was in trouble. I just accepted what was happening as if it was normal and soon went back to bed.

At approximately 4 a.m., I went back to bed but for the next few hours my sleeping pattern was all over the place. I didn't exactly have nightmares but saw lots of scrambled pictures in my head. The silence in my head was deafening and I didn't seem to be able to hear any normal noises outside of me either. When I did finally wake up I couldn't hear either the wind in the huge one- hundred-year-old pine trees along the driveway outside our window, my baby's crying, or what anyone was saying to me. I had to lip read to understand what was being said to me.

I felt as if I was living in a silent world inhabited only by me. That is, until a few hours later when, what happened the night before paled into insignificance.

A few hours later when I did wake up properly, I felt a bit calmer and started the day as normal by visiting the bathroom and toilet, (one room), and there I was to suffer the biggest and most traumatising grief-filled shock of my life. The mental, physical and emotional events of the night before had shocked and traumatised my system so severely that I lost my unborn baby, sight unseen, straight down the toilet.

I stood there stunned, devastated! Shock had stopped me dead. I must have been about one month pregnant. All I could think about was the loss of my unborn child! My heart hurt so much it felt as though it was breaking, it was the most awful feeling. I hadn't known I was pregnant!

Standing there, I felt myself sinking deeper and deeper into nothingness. The shock at first stopped me feeling anything except my hurting heart. There was only a feeling of emptiness as I realised the attack had not just been a personal attack on me; it had now killed my unborn child.

I couldn't breathe, I thought I was going to be sick; I nearly fainted, but somehow found the strength to continue to stay upright.

Everything felt surreal. My thoughts and actions were again disconnected and I felt separated from reality. I felt as though I was floating up near the ceiling. And as I looked down on myself, I can remember thinking how important being a mother is, and I knew that under normal circumstances, I would always choose to carry a baby to full term. Otherwise, how would I know who he or she really was? Now I would never know. I could hardly breathe, and the pain in my chest made me think I was having a heart attack.

Gradually I calmed down and started to move, but the shock had left me traumatised with a very clear picture in my mind of what had happened emotionally. I felt both disembodied as if I wasn't inside myself, and numb. I walked feeling somehow separated from myself as if I was being followed by a shadow or a ghost. I felt as though there were two of me; one part of me seemed to be walking in the light, the other in the dark.

I had difficulty thinking clearly. Remembering past events was a real challenge. Nothing came naturally. Accessing previously learned behaviours and habits was hard to do. I felt like a child, even though I was nearly thirty years of age. I had to relearn everything. Everything from walking to making and drinking a cup of tea without dropping the cup or missing my mouth when I put the cup up to my lips to drink.

This time, I decided that I should ask for help. I rang our Catholic, male doctor for an appointment. In his office, he listened to my story. Then, without a word, stood up, walked to the surgery door, held it open and said, 'I think you should go home and be a good wife and mother.'

I was stunned to hear what he said! Instantly a picture flashed into my mind of an argument I had had with my parents when they thought I was lying, and I knew that for some reason he thought I was lying. Without a word, he stood there holding the door open waiting for me to leave!

I had no choice but to do as he directed me to do, so I stood up and wobbled out of the surgery. He had offered me no physical examination, no words of advice or understanding and once again I felt that awful feeling of defeat close in on me.

On my way home, I went to the Police Station to see if I could get some help, but it was closed. We were living in a small country town, and I couldn't wait around for it to open because I was needed at home where my baby was waiting to be fed.

This was the seventies, and there was little or no professional help available. I told my family what had happened but no-one believed me so there was no hope of receiving any help or support from them. Rehabilitation after shocking events at that time was left to individuals and their families.

In the next few years, both my parents had strokes. This, of course, put pressure on all our family members, so nothing changed for me even though foolishly I still lived in hope that they would change decades of poor attitudes towards me and care about me. Sometimes we are fools for years!

DREAMS

My life's dream was that I really wanted to be happily married with my own family and, if possible, be the perfect wife, mother, and homemaker. I wanted my family to be the opposite from the one I grew up in. I wanted my family to be loving, supportive and kind and here I was again, having to wear a mask to hide what was happening inside me.

But support from my family was not to be!

Hiding my insecurities stressed my nervous system and my sleeping habits changed. Previously, before the attack, I slept well, but now there were nightmares and I hardly ever slept through the night. Once again, exhaustion took over. Keeping life looking as normal as possible on the outside for others to see was exhausting and headaches and digestion problems, which I had sometimes suffered from when stressed, returned.

People have different ways of dealing with their various levels of stress, anxiety, shock, and trauma. Some people withdraw inside their families as my father did; some take to drink and end up becoming alcoholics and others, like me, keep on moving. But continuing to move at that time did not give me the answers I was looking for and there was still more to overcome.

My husband's next big career move was to Singapore. It was there that another incident profoundly impacted my life. With the pressures and adjustments of moving, it wasn't long before my PTSD symptoms started to reappear and I made an appointment to see a doctor.

I had three appointments with him when he did all the usual blood tests, etc. On the third visit, he said, 'I don't know what is wrong with you, and I suggest that you return home to Australia. If you stay here in Singapore, you will die. I had another patient with the same symptoms as yours, and I sent her back to Canada!'

I could not believe my ears. I went into shock. He was using nearly the same words 'go home' as my local doctor had used years earlier. I heard those fearful words again. Only this time I was living in fear in a foreign country and I had four children whom I loved dearly to care for and protect. And maybe, just maybe, I was going to die!

I asked myself, what am I going to do this time? Quickly my husband and I decided that the only thing we could do was return our family to Australia and that is what we did. After only a short time in Singapore, about five months, we were on the move again.

In fifteen years, we moved about eleven times; at least half of those moves were significant moves within Australia, where we moved from state to state to live in new and unknown cities.

Most of the relocations were necessary career moves for my husband. These moves, however, put tremendous pressure on all of us, mainly because of the stress of the long distances. With each move, we needed to find new homes to live in and new schools to go to. All these demands had to be met while adjusting to weather extremes — either hot or cold climates within Australia. Each move was more exhausting than the previous one, and the worst thing was we were never in one place long enough to make friends, so we were a very lonely and lost family.

CHANGE

By this time, I was in my mid-forties and I knew I was not coping well with the situation I was in. I began to think I was heading for total burnout because I was utterly exhausted from living with the fear that I might die, and constantly worried about what would happen to our children if I did die.

In this confused state of mind, I made the biggest mistake of my life — I filed for divorce and against the advice of the family court, I gave full custody of our children to their father.

I have no excuse for doing this, except to say that because I was so exhausted I really believed, at the time, that I might die. My thoughts and hopes were that our children would eventually adjust to, and benefit from living a steadier life with their father rather than living with the uncertainties of life (or death) with their mother. I also knew their father could afford to look after them and give them a good education which I could not afford.

I thought that if I kept trying to manage everything on my

own our children would end up with no mother at all. I felt that they would adjust to living with their father if something happened to me and I knew that if I survived, I would be there for them anyway.

So, this is my story… the consequences of which I have had to face and live with my entire life. The worst part was watching the huge adjustments my children had to make over the first few years after the divorce. It nearly broke my heart to see how hard it was for them to adjust to living in boarding school in Australia and living with their father whose career meant that he was overseas most of the time.

I had made an enormous legal error, regarding the distribution of power in our family. I was living close to where our children were going to school but I was powerless to help them or make any decisions on their behalf.

Their father had all the power!

Without realising what I had done, I had given their father control over our family as part of the divorce settlement. Handing over control, as I had done, left me with no decision-making power at all, and more critical to growing teenagers, I could not contribute financially to any of their teenage needs. I could only offer them love, care and concern.

I have often been questioned about not fighting for my rights.

First, I needed someone to fight for me, and the solicitor I chose was totally ineffective. Second, divorce is a costly business at any time, but even more so when a spouse is overseas, and I did not have any financial or family backing.

These were difficult times for all of us, and as I tried to create a new identity for me, our children got to see their mother living in the worst circumstances they had ever seen in their lives. Yes, my circumstances were difficult for both me and them to adjust to.

Previously, we were the family of an Airline Pilot. We lived and travelled well! That was the life our children were used to, and now their traumatised mother in her mid-forties was unemployed and living on a minimal income. Thus, we grew away from one another.

A NEW BEGINNING

Trauma Free is the story of my search for answers. First, I wanted to know what was wrong with me and then, I wanted to know how I could heal myself when no-one believed what had happened to me, or even heard my cry for help.

Today help is available. All one needs to do is ask. Start reading, talk to others who can help, or search the Internet for answers.

Scientifically, we can ask for brain scans and MRIs to help with the diagnosis to find out if there is anything physically wrong. And there are psychiatrists, psychologists, and counsellors available to help us deal with the mental and emotional issues of a difficult life.

Some years after I was attacked, I had X-rays taken and was told that there was no physical damage to my head and neck. Physically they said, I was okay but it took me years to learn how to live with my emotional imbalances.

I always lacked self-esteem, and since the attack, I once again had no self-confidence. I kept blaming myself for what happened and believed that on some universal level, I had done something terribly wrong and deserved this 'ugly' life. Feelings of guilt and fear stopped me from really wanting to achieve anything in life just in case once again I attracted similar situations.

I was in my sixties before I really understood just how damaging verbal abuse and past patterns and habits could be and apart from writing this book I felt that, by then, it was too late to make significant changes in my life anyway.

Living in fear is a terrible way to live. I have spoken to many people about fear and trauma, and they all say they feel the same way. Most indicate that they choose to live in the comfort zone they have created for themselves rather than make changes which might cause them to end up experiencing a higher level of PTSD and fear, even if the comfort zone they have chosen to live in is not a successful or perfect one.

In my traumatised state, I did not know where to go to ask for help, or, what questions to ask when I got there. Most of the time there was a continuous dialogue in my mind which I could not stop, and I still had lots of sleep and digestion problems

I felt as though I was going out of my mind, and worst of all, I could not get rid of the single pictures (like on a mobile phone) that were also in my mind. Pictures of the many shocks I had suffered. Pictures of both my sister's brush with death and my own shocks were still there as clear as when they happened.

BREAKTHROUGH

I did, at one time, tell our family doctor some of what I felt when I took one of our children to get an immunization injection. The next time I went to visit him, with one of the children, he said he had given some thought to my problem and suggested that I could admit myself voluntarily into Kew Mental Hospital, near Melbourne, Australia for a weekend or two.

I hadn't told the local doctor much about myself, and I did not expect any help, but he had listened anyway and was the first and only person to attempt to offer me professional help.

I questioned taking his advice which seemed to me to be such drastic action because I thought the doctor was implying that I was mentally unstable. At the time, I figured I was managing life reasonably well. However, when I thought about his advice, I knew that voluntarily admitting myself into the mental hospital he had mentioned was the right thing to do.

So, in the early 1970s, I checked myself into the mental

hospital which was near where we were living. One of my best decisions, thankfully, it only took two sessions for me to discover one of the answers I was looking for.

My treatment consisted of being given a drug of some sort that caused me to hallucinate about my sister's brush with death. I saw a picture in my mind's eye of my sister coughing, and I knew immediately that somehow her brush with death and my near-death experience were connected even though they occurred twenty years apart. Both incidents took place on farms, and both left me feeling sick and powerless.

I felt so much better as a glimmer of hope entered my mind and the chattering in my mind eased off for a while. I didn't know it at the time but at last, I had found part of the answer I was looking for. I did not understand all of what had happened during the sessions but left there feeling that some of the heavy emotional burden I was carrying had been lifted off me and more importantly I left there knowing I wasn't mental. I had a clean bill of health and did not need another appointment, they said.

I was far from being healed, but the breakthrough of realising that the pictures and the feelings may be connected was positive. It was, however, many years before I started on my own healing path and quite some time before I understood how the nervous system and the subconscious and conscious minds work together with emotions and pictures when collecting and recording information, and it was decades before I fully understood and recognised what I had done when I mentally stored away those *pictures* and their attached *emotional feelings* in my mind.

At that time, however, I experienced relief as my panic breathing slowed down and my adrenaline, (and fear), subsided. I felt peaceful and relaxed for the first time in ages. Knowledge had given me a feeling of relief and unbeknown to me I had subconsciously, by making the connection between the pictures and emotions filed away in my subconscious, gained the information I would need in the 1990s to start developing 'Trauma Therapy'.

Seeing the 'picture', in my mind's eye, of the shock I suffered when my sister nearly died, and gaining the knowledge that the connection between the two major shocks in my life had an emotional basis didn't fully heal me. More work was needed before that could happen, but it stopped me from feeling nauseated every time I drove into a farming environment. I was still traumatised, and we were still living on our farm and that at times still triggered the symptoms of my own PTSD, but I was able to keep these symptoms hidden and under control.

The panicky feelings connected with trauma, the difficulty breathing, quivering on the inside, shaking on the outside, feeling anxious when I was near my own children, or far away from them, were frightening feelings that made my day-to-day living very difficult, and fear and adrenaline continued to drive my nervous system leaving me feeling exhausted.

The intervening years between subconsciously filing away the information I needed to develop 'Trauma Therapy' were long and lonely mainly because I was the only one doing the work on developing 'Trauma Therapy'.

These days I know, however, that it takes only a short time to get good results from using and understanding 'Trauma Therapy', but it took me years to learn what to do; and do it.

In thinking about both 'farm' incidents, I realised that the first shock was objective. It was about my sister, not about me. I was only indirectly affected. Therefore, it had a less traumatic effect on me, and the PTSD symptoms were less.

The second shock, however, was subjective; it was all about me, my family and my domestic situation.

I was the one directly impacted. I was the one left chronically traumatised and it was only when I realised that PTSD has varying levels of severity that I began asking the right questions of myself.

How could I bring peace into my life permanently?

How did it happen that I felt so relieved when I found the picture connection?

What had I discovered when I saw the picture?

Why was my domestic scenario continuing to negatively impact me?

Could I further help myself by also dealing with the many shocks I had experienced up to that time and most interesting of all could I help others heal themselves? My issues of co-dependency concerning helping others were deeply embedded in me, but maybe this time helping them would help me, maybe helping them would work for me, instead of against me.

The main question was — what is the common denominator, what is it that links everything together? I said to myself over, and over again, there must be another key to unlock the puzzle of the symptoms of PTSD. Looking at PTSD symptoms as I understood them was getting me nowhere. But what was the key? They implied a mental disorder and I knew I wasn't mental.

1994 was the magic year!

Previously I had already written, self-published, and later published, "Natural Stress and Anxiety Relief." *How to*

Use the Johnson Breathing Technique. The Adrenaline Connection. www.amazon.com In it, I explain in detail how the body's adrenaline-driven *fight or flight* response to shock affects the nervous system. I also discuss how, by using the correct muscles to breathe with, we can start to control adrenaline and slow the nervous system down so that the physical body can stop the constant not always needed flow of adrenaline.

When the body runs on adrenaline, it alters how the body functions, e.g., nervous system, digestion, sleep patterns, etc. Dropping the adrenaline level helps to stop the body developing an adrenaline addiction, and this, in turn, helps the body and mind stay calm and healthy. Adrenaline is the right response for fight or flight, but not for everyday living.

Understanding how adrenaline and breathing directly affect the body and health was, however, not the entire answer for me.

I needed more information.

I knew how to breathe correctly and was reasonably healthy, but I also knew I was not quite as healthy as I would like to be. I was, for instance, still very tired.

Adding 'Trauma Therapy' to my understanding of the damage adrenaline addiction caused helped me break through my own 'fear' barrier. It helped me gradually answer all the questions I was still asking me and this in turn helped me find and release the true me.

1994

In 1994, I was visiting a friend who knew about the work I was doing. Feeling safe in her home and with her permission, while she was making dinner, I decided to delve into that fearful place inside me where my *emotional feeling words* were hidden.

Breaking through my own fear barrier on my own was the scariest thing I have ever had to do. But suddenly the breakthrough came, and I saw a *picture* of the terrible scene I had lived through when I was attacked. I concentrated on the clear *picture* in my mind's eye of the attack and using the format of 'Trauma Therapy', identified the attached *emotional feeling word* which was connected to the *'picture'* and quickly released it.

The word was 'terrified' and terrified I had been.

After a good, restful night's sleep, I went into the bathroom the next morning and had visual proof that the trauma was released. There, just above my collarbones, at the base of my neck were four round black bruises slightly smaller than the size of golf balls. I called my friend in to see what had happened, and she was as amazed as I was with the proof that was so obvious. It showed clearly that 'Trauma Therapy' worked. Here was clear evidence that I had released the shock, terror and internalised bruising of that dreadful night. I didn't just feel calmer and different that next morning I also absolutely knew I could now start to heal all the other shocks that had affected my life.

I was traumatised, mentally, physically and emotionally from being physically attacked, and, terribly hurt and bruised by the ignorance and thoughtlessness of others when seeking their love, kindness, empathy, understanding, and support but now that I knew 'Trauma Therapy' really worked, I had work to do. Now I could stop feeling sorry for myself and do something positive to effect change. Now I could really start healing myself.

In doing the work on myself, I slowly began to release the truth of my 'ugly' life. I have asked myself many times, was it a preordained program of ugliness I was born with, did I create the program myself or did others program me into who I am. The answer — Who knows?

At no time did I want to blame anyone as might be expected. Remember I was conditioned to turn the other cheek, from the beginning and that was strong conditioning. But, when the time came as it did for me to recognise what I could do to help myself that is exactly what I did. I turned away from the people who had hurt me and started helping myself to heal. It was good for me to recognise the truth because then, and only then, was I able to first, accept myself as I was and second accept change and work with it.

CHANGES

In the years that followed, I observed changes in myself. They were subtle changes at first. I always blamed myself for the failure I was, but gradually I began to see that all of life is about interacting with others and I soon realised that some of what I had gone through was the fault of others. But not once in all those years did I really blame anyone else except myself for my challenges, and labels such as 'emotional abuse' and 'domestic violence' were unheard of in those days so there was no way of me describing to myself or anyone else what had happened, and was happening to me.

My church and religious teachings in my early years had taught me well. I was to turn the other cheek when others did wrong by me. Those teachings conditioned me to not show my feelings, not fight back and not ask for help.

It was only when I decided to let go of some of my emotional pain, stop feeling sorry for myself and start taking responsibility for my life that everything began to work out for me.

I could now see the truth of my situation, and what I had become; there was two sides to my story, and at last, I knew I was not totally to blame — what a relief!

I had stopped vaguely blaming others years ago for seeming to have the wrong attitudes and behaviours towards me because life had taught me that most of the answers I sought were inside me. Sharing some of the blame for feeling like a failure in life did, thankfully, lift some of my powerfully destructive shame and guilt feelings.

Suddenly awakening to the fact that I could see where other's attitudes and behaviours had affected me was a great relief. Understanding the truth of where the blame lay, in my disappointingly 'ugly' failure of a life, had somehow freed me and I now took on board the truth that it takes two to create any situation. I still asked myself was the programming there from the very beginning and other rather negative unanswerable questions — who knows? Sometimes we do not always have all the answers, and that is also okay.

'Trauma Therapy' was my truth. Gradually over time, I recognised what needed to be done to acknowledge my truth. As I did the work on myself, I released myself from many of the frustrations of the past.

Thus, I would like to say to anyone who has suffered — believe in you. Keep searching, and you will find your answers.

I searched about looking for answers, when all the time they were inside me, not outside of me in other places. A school motto I know of says it all, Vincit Qui Se Vincit — She Conquers Who Conquers Herself. That truly was the truth for me, the answers were inside me all the time, and when I found the courage, time, and patience I needed to use 'Trauma Therapy' on myself, I found even more of my own truthful answers. They were inside me!

My journey has been a lonely one, but I had magnificent friends whom I thank from the bottom of my heart. I did most of the work developing 'Trauma Therapy' and healed myself, but I could not have done it without the love and support of my friends.

This book is about helping! I do know now that — **it is never too late!**

If you are traumatised, do something about your PTSD. It does not matter what level of PTSD you are suffering from, all you need to do is ask yourself, 'do I have a picture in my mind's eye of a bad experience I have suffered through'? If you have a picture, you have something to work with. All you need to do is recognise that you have a picture to work with and release it using the 'five steps' of 'Trauma Therapy'.

Release your shock and ease your trauma. Help yourself by releasing the *emotional feeling words* connected to the original shock, e.g., *'picture,'* or *'pictures.'* There may be many pictures. Take your time and work with each one.

We all have the capacity to help ourselves and others. All we need to do is stop and think, and become mindful of what it is we really want out of life. I wanted to understand more about myself and live a more peaceful and happy family life — what is it you really want?

I have found many of my answers, and my PTSD umbrella now stands behind the front door, its wings are folded, and it is peaceful, as am I.

No-one is immune! Shock and trauma do not discriminate; anyone can be affected:

- Children who live in a household where PTSD has altered their way of life in some way, e.g., illness, altered behaviours, and attitudes, etc.

- Veterans, peacekeepers, and families who may still be affected by subsequent wars, e.g., Vietnam

- Emergency services such as Police, Fire and Ambulance and their families

- Teachers who have been verbally or physically abused at school

- Abused parents

- Abused children — incest victims, victims of abusive parenting

- Traumatised victims from the World Trade Centre collapse, Pandemics — Coronavirus (COVID-19) and Epidemics who feel as though their lives are still off balance

- Families who have lost their homes, e.g., bushfires, flooding, typhoons, nuclear disasters

- Those family members who are left behind in shock after airplane crashes

- Car accidents

- Anyone who has suffered a shock, is traumatised or has a picture to work with

- Many health problems can be affected by PTSD. Depression, chronic fatigue and burnout are but a few. Many other illnesses are mentioned throughout this book — *Trauma Free, Your Five Steps to Freedom.*

AUTHORS NOTE

In developing 'Trauma Therapy', I have substituted the words flashback and flashbacks, words which are used by some other areas of trauma counselling, with the words picture and pictures.

The word flashback can be intimidating, because as soon as it is used it causes people to 'flash' instantly 'back' into their scary and/or frightening past where they relive, mentally, physically and emotionally the original situation that caused their shock and subsequent trauma — their PTSD.

Reliving the past, therefore, perpetuates the trauma cycle.

Substituting the words picture and pictures stops emotional regression. This helps clients stay focused on the picture of the original incident. It keeps them in the present; in the here and now and helps them break the cycle of regressing into the feelings of their emotionally charged past, empowering them, if the 'Therapy' works, into feeling that here, at last, is help they can trust.

As you will see in the following pages, there are times when other therapies could and should be chosen. 'Trauma Therapy', like any other form of counselling, is not for everyone. It is always wise to consider discussing with your therapist or health care worker whether 'Trauma Therapy' is suitable for you.

PART II
Trauma Therapy

Trauma is the physical, mental and emotional condition that affects the body and mind when the nervous system suffers an emotional shock. Trauma, now called Post-Traumatic Stress Disorder, (PTSD) is a condition which can be difficult to diagnose, treat and heal.

Trauma Free, Your Five Steps to Freedom offers a simple explanation about how to diagnose and treat PTSD, (trauma). Another book I have written and published focuses on how adrenaline as an addiction affects the body. It suggests ways of identifying and managing stress, anxiety and other health problems which may be linked to the addiction of adrenaline.

'Natural Stress and Anxiety Relief'. *How to Use the Johnson Breathing Technique. The Adrenaline Connection* is available from www.amazon,com. It is the lead up to what I have written about in this book in both knowledge and understanding.

Both books: 'Natural Stress and Anxiety Relief' and, 'Trauma Free', acknowledge the distress caused to the nervous system and the mind and body when they are affected by shock and adrenaline.

Shocks which have many causes pre-empt trauma.

Good shocks are few in number, they may include suddenly winning lotto; or, a much sought- after trophy, or, receiving good news, etc. Bad or adverse shocks are many in number and their causes may include being in a car accident, abuse, domestic violence, war, hearing of the sudden death of a loved one, or, that a much-needed operation is imminent, etc.

Shock and trauma are connected and are recognised by the fact that they concern remembered events.

MOST PEOPLE REMEMBER THESE EVENTS EASILY, AND HAVE A CLEAR PICTURE IN THEIR MIND'S EYE CONNECTED TO THE EVENT OR INCIDENT THAT CAUSED THEIR SHOCK. THESE PICTURES ARE LINKED TO STRONG EMOTIONAL FEELINGS; FEELINGS THAT ARE RECORDED AND REMEMBERED IN THE MIND FROM THE TIME OF THE ORIGINAL EVENT, I.E., THE ORIGINAL SHOCK.

Shocks cause people to feel 'different'! Sometimes they feel separated or disconnected in some way from themselves, others or their surroundings.

HOW DOES SEPARATION OR DISCONNECT HAPPEN?

Separation/disconnection happens at the moment of shock when the body's automatic natural survival system activates.

The body when it experiences shock automatically takes a big breath, panic breathes, high in the chest, triggering adrenaline.

As this happens, (1) physically a person's breathing changes, (2) the mind takes a photo of what is happening at the moment of shock, (3) the mind records whatever emotion a person is feeling at that precise moment. Technically how the mind does this I do not know. What I do know, however, is that instantly at the moment of shock the conscious and subconscious minds work together but separately as they record what is happening. The conscious mind sees what is happening in the present and the subconscious mind automatically records and remembers the event and the internalised feeling word. If natural reconnection does not immediately follow a shock, then the body and mind become confused and trauma follows. This leaves a person in a traumatised state not knowing how to think clearly and behave; they *feel* not quite right, not normal, as if there is something wrong, but not knowing what it is that is wrong.

The longer this feeling of disconnection continues, the harder it is to reconnect. If reconnection does not occur instantly, trauma follows, its symptoms increasing in severity as time goes by.

Because of our natural inbuilt automatic survival response most people adjust to life after a shock. They continue to live their 'normal' lives. They do this by automatically drawing on previously learned habits already stored in the subconscious. They may, however, find that they need to learn new habits if they are traumatised and disconnected. Knowing how to release the internalised emotional feeling word allows the body and mind to return to normal.

'Trauma Therapy', the therapy I developed to treat my own trauma focuses on releasing the internalised emotional feeling word and can be used by both, a trained therapist, or an untrained person. Here, in this book, my dialogue is written from the point of view of the trained therapist. In later pages there is a dialogue an untrained person can read through.

THE KEY TO THE SUCCESS OF 'TRAUMA THERAPY' IS THAT THE THERAPIST FOLLOWING THE GUIDELINES OF 'TRAUMA

Therapy' works with the client's agenda, not the therapist's agenda. The client and therapist dialogue together following the five questions and answers of the format of 'Trauma Therapy'.

'Trauma Therapy' is about a client's internalised *pictures* and *emotional feeling words* concerning the event or incident that caused them to suffer a shock. It is not about what the therapist thinks happened to the client. A client has his/her own unique answers and knows what emotional feeling word/words they internalised at the instant of shock. Using the structured principles of 'Trauma Therapy', when questioned, clients will reveal their own answers. These will be the correct answers for the client.

Sometimes a client will fail to identify an emotional feeling word. If this happens, there are two reasons why a trained therapist will get results more quickly when helping their clients identify the emotional feeling word attached to the picture recorded in the mind.

One reason for this difference is that, with practice, a trained therapist has already learned how to observe every nuance of their client's, physical behaviour e.g. hand movements, facial expressions, body and eye movements. The other reason for the difference in quality of work and therefore results, may be because the therapist is trained to listen carefully to what the client is saying when telling his/her story and is therefore able to pick up on, and label whatever the underlying emotion is.

Generally, issues are resolved one at a time. There is one shock, but there may be many emotional feeling words relating to that one shock or issue. To get the best results all emotional feeling words need to be identified and released.

Each and every one of us who has suffered, or is suffering from the effects of a shock, called trauma, (PTSD), has within us the answers to the questions a therapist will ask. **THE THERAPIST'S ROLE, WHEN USING 'TRAUMA THERAPY', IS TO DIRECTLY ENABLE CLIENTS FIND THEIR OWN ANSWERS.**

The principles of how to use 'Trauma Therapy' are specific and closed questions are used more often than in other models of counselling. Closed questions are specific questions which require a 'yes' or 'no' answer, rather than a longer answer which can turn into a discussion. In 'Trauma Therapy' there is no need for a discussion because closed questions elicit the short 'yes' or 'no' answers needed.

Times for discussion are either before or after using 'Trauma Therapy'.

THERE ARE SAFETY NETS FOR BOTH CLIENT AND THERAPIST.

First, the client has control of what issues they want to work on.

Initially, clients are asked two questions — one question is, have you ever suffered a shock, and the other question is, do you have a picture in your mind's eye of the incident that caused the shock? Mostly clients answer, 'yes' to both questions and are quite surprised to realise they can see a picture of the incident. There will be only one picture at a time in the mind's eye. The therapist may think that the client has chosen the wrong picture but the client knows best and that picture is the one they must work with.

Second, 'Trauma Therapy' is a thinking therapy where the client and therapist interact intellectually. Clients are encouraged to remain mindful and focused in present time, thinking about what is happening in the here and now rather than going down into their feelings and emotions when addressing past issues.

Clients, in staying centred and present, experience less emotional stress and anxiety when addressing past issues.

Most clients tell me they feel happier using a thinking model of therapy rather than continuing to be emotionally traumatised by repeatedly going back over past issues.

Working in this way gives clients a feeling of being in 'control'. They also have a sense of trust and feel more secure because they feel as though the therapist really wants to help, is listening to them, and is willing to work with them at their own pace with their own personal issues. Anyone who has been a client in an unsuccessful counselling session will relate to these thoughts because of the 'uncomfortable' feelings they experienced when they thought they were not being heard.

THE FOLLOWING IS AN OVERVIEW OF A STRAIGHTFORWARD 'TRAUMA THERAPY' SESSION

A client, a businessman in his thirties, presented to me with what he and I both thought were unresolved anger issues concerning his father. I observed that he was very restless. He couldn't sit still and kept on talking about his father as he squeezed his hands together.

Before he felt safe enough to choose a 'picture' to work with, a picture that would allow him to get near his very powerful, controlling, and frightening feeling of anger, he needed to work with his stress and anxiety, and his adrenaline addiction. He had some resistance to dealing with his stress because he thought it was not his problem, but eventually realised that he needed to stop running on adrenaline and calm his nervous system down a little before he could concentrate on using 'Trauma Therapy' successfully.

At first, when I asked him to recall a picture of an interaction with his father, instead of being able to think about the past without getting angry, he came back to the present and current issues. After showing him how to calm his nervous system so that he could control his adrenaline, stress and anxiety, I was able to help him concentrate on what he had to do to effectively work with ' Trauma Therapy'.

He found it much easier to concentrate on what was required of him when he was calmer.

The picture he chose to work with was one of him at age nine. He saw and remembered the incident clearly.

He remembered his father blaming him for something he did not do. In the scene, his father was furious and would not listen to any reasoning from his son. My client said he could remember feeling powerless and angry at the time, and he knew he had 'swallowed' his anger. He also remembered feeling frightened of how angry his father was.

On completing the exercise he released his emotional feeling word, anger. At the same time he realised that what he had internalised about his father at the time of the incident probably caused him to have low self-esteem. He said he always had great difficulty speaking up for himself, (swallowed anger), where his father and other males were concerned — especially in the business world and thoughtfully added that being stuck back in the past feeling angry and thinking negative thoughts could probably be the reason why he lacked self-esteem.

He also recognised that many other decisions he had made throughout his life were based on other spontaneous thoughts and feelings he had internalised at that time, and other times. These included the feeling of fear. This feeling of fear stopped him from being able to speak up for himself, and more importantly, he internalised a statement which said, 'I hate my father and don't want to be a *man* like him!' Thinking statements like that made him feel insignificant as though he had no (male) self-esteem, he said.

He sat there with a look of stunned amazement on his face and admitted sheepishly that he came to see me thinking that anger was his only problem. He said he had always feared his father, and now he knew why. Fear, he said, was behind his anger, fear made it difficult for him to speak up for himself and make, what others would typically say were 'male' decisions. Decisions such as, what type of work he would do when he left school.

Fear also stopped him from having healthy relationships with both men and women, but especially with men. What a relief, he said with a big sigh, as his body sagged and he relaxed.

The one word he released was — anger. He realised that he was justified in feeling the way he did about his father. His judgment of his father was correct. His father was wrong to behave badly in front of his son. He said thoughtfully, 'knowing I was right in my judgment back then should help me make better decisions in the future.' I agreed with him and added that because he completed the exercise successfully, he should also feel more empowered when making male-related decisions in the future. The session helped him understand the damage powerful, unresolved feelings had caused in his life. One picture, one emotional feeling word!

My client validated himself. He didn't need me to do it for him and left the clinic feeling and looking happier, calmer and much more relaxed.

I saw him for a few more sessions to reinforce the breathing technique I had taught him so that he could control his adrenaline, stress and anxiety. It took a while for him to get the breathing technique right and get used to the idea that he could do both — stay calm, and make his own good decisions. At one stage, he said to me, 'I need to practise making decisions,' I agreed with him!

We discussed other changes he would need to make, and I reminded him that, like all things new, it would take a while to control his adrenaline addiction, change his past habits and learn what to do to act differently in the present to get his future needs met.

INDICATIONS FOR USING 'TRAUMA THERAPY' ARE WHEN A CLIENT SAYS:

a) 'I can't get this picture/s out of my mind ...'

b) 'I can remember when ...'

c) 'My life has not been the same since ...'

d) 'I feel disconnected from the person I used to be.'

e) 'I'm not the same person since the death of my mother, spouse, operation or accident,' etc.

f) 'I can't stop my mind from running on.'

g) 'I have not felt the same since ...'

h) 'I feel angry all the time.'

Example

One day, another of my clients, a young mother with a child of three arrived looking tired and harassed. She sat down suddenly and said to me that she had *'not felt the same since'* the birth of her little boy and the death of her grandmother who died two days after the birth of her great-grandson.

The mother and grandmother lived in the same city, but

were, at the time of the birth, in different hospitals. Both had a very close relationship with each other; but, because the baby's birth had been a difficult one, the nursing staff and the woman's relatives took 'control' of the situation and advised her not to get out of bed to go visit her grandmother. She therefore never had closure with the passing of her grandmother, and was unfortunately unable to show her newborn to his great-grandmother.

She said she felt as though she was being controlled by others. She said that she could no longer make decisions, and if she did, she couldn't follow through with them.

These surface issues seemed to be connected to normal grief and loss issues. One issue that of not being able to show her new baby to someone special, and the other issue, of not being able to say goodbye to that same special person before she died. Consequently she had been helped to deal with her grief and loss issues through months of counselling and was happy with the results.

As I listened to her, I had my own internal dialogue going. I observed her hand movements and thought to myself, there are other issues and emotional feeling words that should be recognised and released here. I thought of words such as anger, control, frustration, and powerlessness. I did not say anything to the client and that was wise because the outcome after choosing to use 'Trauma Therapy' was entirely different from what I had expected it would be.

It was not words like anger, control, frustration, and powerlessness, which she identified and released. But, the word 'confused.' She had disconnected from herself, in shock when others took control i.e., when others stopped her from making her own decisions. Since then she had not reconnected and thereafter felt very confused.

This young woman had been in control of her decision making processes before her baby was born was now disconnected, traumatised and unable to access her normal decision-making skills, and now felt as though she had lost *control* of her life.

Everyone else made decisions for her, concerning her grandmother, at a critical time in her life, and she now felt powerless to make efficient, sound decisions herself.

After being accustomed to being in control of her life, and making her own decisions, the shock of others taking the control away from her caused her to go into shock and disconnect from her previously learned, normal, focused, decision-making self. It left her feeling confused and traumatised. Even though she intellectually understood that the decisions made on her behalf, at the hospital were the right ones, she hadn't since reconnected after the shock of being told what to do and hadn't since reverted back to the habit of making good decisions easily. She had simply let others make her decisions for her at the time, and she was still letting others make her decisions for her because she felt too confused to make them for herself.

By following the 'Trauma Therapy' format, my client identified and released the word 'confused', her emotional feeling word.

When she came back to see me a week later, she was a different person. She said she felt euphoric and more important than feeling happy, she could think clearly, make decisions, and follow through on them. The feeling of confusion had gone.

She thanked me for using a thinking therapy to help her release her emotional feeling word. She said that she felt as though she understood more clearly what was happening during the session and later admitted that she hadn't wanted to go back over her past history. She said that using a thinking model of therapy gave her a feeling of being in 'control' during the session.

This session, once again, reminded me that the therapist's role is an empathic, nonjudgmental role when using 'Trauma Therapy'.

I ALSO REMINDED MYSELF THAT EACH AND EVERY PERSON HAS THEIR OWN ANSWERS IF THEY HAVE A PICTURE TO WORK WITH.

'TRAUMA THERAPY'

THE EXERCISE AND HOW TO USE IT WHEN YOUR CLIENT SAYS — 'YES', TO THE QUESTION OF:

'DO YOU HAVE A PICTURE TO WORK WITH?'

If, after you have listened to your client's story, you think you do not have enough information, ask a few more questions to clarify exactly what they are talking about, then when you are satisfied that you have enough information continue with the session using 'Trauma Therapy'.

'TRAUMA THERAPY' — EXERCISE FORMAT:

This example of a 'Trauma Therapy' session may help both trained and untrained persons understand the usefulness and impact of 'Trauma Therapy'.

a) Ask your client if they have a picture in their

mind's eye connected with their shock. Most clients will answer 'yes'. Ask them if their picture is like those taken with a mobile/cell phone. The picture chosen to work with must be a still picture like those taken on a mobile/cell phone.

b) Clarify whether your client has ever had a nickname or been called by any other first name. In the example, for this exercise, the client's name will be Jan.

Jan rang and made an appointment. She was suffering from ongoing back and neck pain from a car accident ten years earlier. She was driving and had been medically diagnosed as suffering severe whiplash. Having had lots of treatment, both medical and non-medical in the intervening years, she was exhausted from coping with the pain, the many visits she was making to practitioners, and from taking various recommended medications that did not seem to be working.

c) After listening to her story, I asked Jan if she had a picture of the accident in her mind's eye. She said, **'Yes.'** I asked her to 'hold' the picture and focus on it. The picture she chose to work with related exactly to the time of impact. The picture could have, however, related to some other incident, either before, during, or after the accident — for her, it was the accident.

d) I said to her, 'If you look carefully at the picture do you see yourself?' She answered, **'Yes,'** in a surprised voice. Explain to your client that they are looking at the scene as it happened, that they may be facing away from themselves in the picture. Therapists are advised here not to linger too long discussing the picture with clients because some clients will argue that they cannot see themselves at the time of the incident.

If clients want an explanation about what happened to them at the time of the incident explain to them that to protect them at the moment of impact the body automatically goes into shock and activates its adrenaline- driven survival system. The shock causes the mind, (like a camera), to remember a clear picture of the incident. The mind also internalises at the same time an emotional feeling word which describes what a person felt at the time of the incident or accident.

e) If clients are hesitant, reassure them that hesitancy is a normal reaction. Tell them that you are going to run a dialogue with them to help them release the emotional feeling word. Explain to them, that you want them to talk directly to the person in the picture, in their mind's eye — the person who is really him/herself.

f) Ask them to say the words silently to themselves, not aloud. They converse with their inner self, the self who has the answers.

g) Then ask them to say to the person in the picture, **'Is your name Jan?'** Repeat this. Say this aloud so that they understand the framing of the question, **'Is your name Jan?'** (This is a closed question which requires a single answer, either a yes or a no answer). Clients are amazed when the person in the picture answers, **'yes'.** You have now caught their attention and they are ready to continue.

Clients sometimes need to be reassured that they can trust the process. Reassure them again that they are okay and gently ask them to continue with the exercise.

Please Note: Explain to your client that the work is simple and straightforward and that if we are interrupted, we will stop what we are doing and continue with the exercise after the interruption. Tell them that sometimes there are unavoidable interruptions such as the phone ringing or someone knocking on the door, etc.

h) Continue by asking Jan to say to the Jan in the picture **'what are you feeling?'** When Jan has had time to ask the question the therapist asks her what Jan said. She answers the therapist with an emotional feeling word. For Jan, her word was, **'pain'**.

i) To help Jan release the negative emotional feeling word 'pain', I then ask her to say to her inner self, **'it is okay to feel pain, but would you like to let the feeling of pain go?'** She answers, **'Yes.'** (The answer is usually, yes.) Then I e.g. ask her to say to her inner self, **'come, walk towards me integrate with me. <u>Stop</u> feeling pain, <u>start</u> relaxing'**. Keep it simple if you can but reinforce and reframe what you have just said if you need to, e.g., **'Let the feeling of pain go, start feeling calm and relaxed so that the healing process can begin.'** (Keep these sentences as short as possible. The subconscious takes everything literally; therefore, the wording needs to be simple, e.g., Stop and Start are simple, easy to understand words).

j) Usually, the client visibly relaxes and when asked if their neck pain has gone, will answer, 'yes' or give a description of what is happening, i.e., my neck and shoulders are much less stressed and painful, although there is still some stiffness. Sometimes the pain does go in one session; at other times it lingers on, and other sessions are needed. This often depends on the level of trauma, how long the pain has been there, what treatments the client has had previously and whether the client internalised other emotional feeling words at the time of the incident; these words will also need to be identified and released.

k) The therapist then waits patiently for the client to relax. For some clients, this can be quite cathartic, although not scary.

l) Their reaction might be that they take a deep releasing breath, calm down and look relaxed. Then, when asked how they feel, they usually say they feel a great sense of relief, the pain has gone, they feel as if a burden has been lifted. Others cry with the relief of letting go, and still, others sit there looking relieved and relaxed, with the biggest smiles on their faces. Most people respond positively to the experience.

Please note: Always check the success of your work. Ask your client 'has the picture gone?' If it has gone, the work is successful. If it has not gone, then more 'Trauma Therapy' is needed. Some pictures have two or three emotional feeling words connected to them. Finally ask your client, 'Do you feel warm somewhere in your body?' Usually, the answer is, yes! If more work is needed, it can be done right then or in another session.

Sometimes I have found when using 'Trauma Therapy' that even though the shock is released and the effect of trauma decreases over time, the damage to the physical body may not change very much. Letting the shock go usually brings a feeling of relief. If there is no relief after using 'Trauma Therapy', alternative treatments should be sought.

In many areas of our lives and work, there is some form of resistance and clinician work is no different. There are always some clients who do not want to change. These people will resist any kind of treatment.

Even though 'Trauma Therapy' is a simple, easy to understand and follow therapy some clients still want to keep their past patterns. They may have a vested interest in keeping their habits and patterns alive, e.g., for attention and/or getting their needs met in some other area. Also, some people are very stubborn; they do not like being told what to do.

If there is resistance, the therapist, especially an experienced therapist, helps the client with a dialogue which gives the inner person a chance to choose whether they want to change, integrate or stay where they are — stuck in the past! The therapist should always remember that the decision to change or not to change is the client's, not the therapist's.

Most clients quickly realise that the 'pictures' and the internalised 'emotional feeling words' have equal importance.

Emotional feeling words can be positive or negative words. Positive emotional feeling words include words such as love, warm, strong, happy, warmth, control, etc. Negative emotional feeling words include words such as — chaos, terrified, paralysed, fright, frightened, guilty, ashamed, humiliated, etc.

Other examples of negative and positive emotional feeling words are mentioned throughout the book.

'Trauma Therapy', THE THERAPY AND HOW TO USE IT WHEN YOUR CLIENT SAYS 'NO' TO THE QUESTION: 'DO YOU HAVE A PICTURE TO WORK WITH?'

If your client, when asked whether they have a picture in their mind's eye to work with answers 'no,' then ask them how they remember the incident. Some will say they just 'do' remember and there is no picture. Others will realise for the first time that they do use pictures to help them remember. Some clients do not understand that they remember with the aid of pictures and are really surprised when they concentrate and see a picture of the actual incident in their mind's eye.

If the client gives a 'no' answer, the therapist needs to listen carefully to what the client is saying when they tell their story. Most clients will eventually say something which indicates that they do have a picture to work with. They will use a visual word, e.g., see, clear, light, dark, etc. when describing what happened.

If there is no picture, and, in fact, the client truly believes there is no picture, then there is a possibility that it may have been blocked from the clients reality because of the very powerful feelings associated with the shock of what was happening at the time of the incident, e.g., terror, anger, fear, hurt, pain, etc.

If the answer is no and the therapist cannot help them find

a picture then the therapist should proceed with their usual, longer counselling session.

CLINICAL EXPERIENCE REGARDING A 'NO' ANSWER TO THE QUESTION OF SEEING A PICTURE

A well-known hypnotist who lived in my area called and made an appointment to see me. As soon as I heard his name, I felt really intrigued as to why he wanted an appointment.

On arrival, he went straight to his reason for being there. The first thing he said was, I cannot remember or see pictures when I think about the past and, indeed, when I talked with him, I realised that what he said was true.

Immediately, for me, the word 'intrigued' turned into the thought, 'I wonder if I will be able to help him?'

Straight away, in telling his story, he went to a time when his father was very angry, frightening him by yelling at him in an outraged voice because he thought his son had done something wrong; his son, however, knew he had done nothing wrong.

I asked my client if he had a picture of the incident in his mind's eye, he answered, 'no.' So I asked him to go through the story again in detail, and carefully watched his eye movements, his facial expressions, and his hand movements. I was looking for a visual clue, rather than listening to the words he was using. At one point his eyes suddenly moved sideways and down. As this happened, I asked him to stop his dialogue, and said to him, 'what did you see as you described that scene.' He looked at me with a surprised expression on his face and said, 'I saw a one-shot picture of my father yelling at me.'

Instantly he realised, where he had lost the ability to see and remember in pictures. He said that, at the time of the confrontation with his father, he felt terrified and hated seeing his father yelling at him. He already knew because of his own work that the mind had a very powerful way of blocking out what it did not want to remember, issues such as fearful episodes just like the one he had lived through. He recognised straight away that he was very scared and added, 'now I know why I became a hypnotherapist!' Hypnosis is about the artificial production of a state resembling deep sleep, in which the subject acts only on external suggestion. This is a way of using suggestions so that a person can access their deepest fears.

My client had been a hypnotherapist for many years and probably started looking for his answer a long time ago. The word fear was his emotional feeling word.

We finished the exercise using the picture he had in his mind's eye and suddenly he could see many pictures, ones he did not know were there, ones that had been blocked and hidden for years.

He sat up straight beaming from ear-to-ear and looking very happy thanked me for opening up a whole new world to him. PLEASE NOTE: **HYPNOSIS IS ABOUT THE ARTIFICIAL PRODUCTION OF A STATE RESEMBLING DEEP SLEEP. 'TRAUMA THERAPY' IS ABOUT BEING FULLY CONSCIOUS, AWAKE AND FOCUSED; TWO ENTIRELY DIFFERENT THERAPIES.**

CHECKING THE SUCCESS OF INTEGRATING 'NEGATIVE' FEELING WORDS

A) **Therapist Observations:** Following is a list of three observations a therapist might look for when assessing the effectiveness of integrating negative feeling words.

- i) When the exercise is successfully completed, the client will take a deep releasing breath like a sigh.

- ii) Clients whose faces looked pale before the exercise often have colour in their faces after the exercise is completed.

- iii) There will be a visible relaxing of the face and body.

B) Client's observations regarding their experience:

i) Clients will say they feel a warm sensation either connected to where the pain was or radiating through their bodies. As the emotional feeling word pain was released in Jan's exercise, the sense of warmth was in her neck and shoulders, although, sometimes it is in other parts of the body as well, (e.g., the centre of the chest, or the legs or hands, etc.).

The radiation of warmth and the release of tension will indicate to you, the therapist, that the therapy has been successful.

ii) Ask your client if they feel lighter. Ask if they feel as if a burden has been lifted. The answer will be in the affirmative and clients will share their own thoughts of what they are experiencing. Generally, there is a positive response; they will say things look brighter. The light itself looks more brilliant, colours are clearer, the trees outside the window look more defined and the feeling of pain is less or gone. Often, they feel less confused.

iii) On the success of the exercise, ask your client if the picture they were working with is still there? If the work has been completed successfully, the answer will be 'no'. At this point, however, do not allow your client to search for the picture. Suggest instead that they concentrate on what we are talking about in the here and now rather than go looking for the picture. I then explain to them that the memory of e.g., the accident or incident is still there, but the picture connected to the shock of what happened could be either gone or lighter. Sometimes the picture is still there but very light, not as defined as it was before which means that more therapy is needed. Whether the neck pain has gone or not, depends on how much more therapy and physical body work, (e.g., massage, physiotherapy), needs to be done.

If, after finishing the therapy your client still has some pain, and their previous reaction to the question about feeling warm somewhere is negative, then go through the exercise again.

Some clients will say the picture is still there, although it is lighter, blurry and less defined than it was before. A therapist will then know that other emotional feeling words, which were internalised at the time of the shock, will also need to be released.

THESE WORDS WILL NEED TO BE IDENTIFIED, RETRIEVED AND RELEASED BY REPEATING THE FORMAT OF 'TRAUMA THERAPY'.

Therapists will observe that clients cooperate with them more easily the second time, having already been through the exercise once.

INTEGRATING POSITIVE — EMOTIONAL FEELING WORDS

Occasionally the 'feeling' you have been working with and the 'picture' your client can see, will not integrate.

If this happens, it may mean that the therapist has concentrated on the emotional feeling word as a 'negative' emotional feeling word, but the client had internalised it as a 'positive' emotional feeling word when they disconnected or separated from themselves at the time of the shock. Positive emotional feeling words are empowering words, e.g., power, motivation, calm, happy, joy, relaxed, love, control, etc.

Positive emotional feeling words are recognised and brought forward in the integration process, whereas ***negative*** emotional feeling words are released, they are let go of! There are fewer positive emotional feeling words than there are negative emotional feeling words and it is important to understand that some words can be either a positive or negative emotional feeling word, e.g., control, power, etc.

On those rare occasions when the client is struggling to find the right word, an experienced therapist will make changes to the 'Trauma Therapy' format wording if they get stuck.

The therapist will encourage, e.g., Jan to say to her inner self — 'my name is also Jan, and you are a part of me that has become separated and stuck in the past.' **Jan then says to her inner self,** 'I have forgotten what it feels like to be in control, (positive feeling word). Would you like to let the past go, integrate with me, come through to where I am now, and share your feeling of being in control with me?'

Generally, the answer to this question is **'yes'.** If the answer is **'yes,'** Jan says, **'come towards me, integrate with me and bring your feeling of control with you so that together we can take control.'**

By this time clients have begun to trust the process for two reasons:
1. They have built up trust with their therapist and,

2. having been through the exercise once they now have some idea of what they are doing.

Clients watch their internal processes with keen interest

especially when they are working with a positive emotional feeling word, like the word 'control'. Clients like the idea of taking back control.

CHECKING THE SUCCESS OF INTEGRATING POSITIVE EMOTIONAL FEELING WORDS –

Therapist and client observations are the same when using either positive or negative emotional feeling words.

Therapist Observations: Following is a repeat list of three observations a therapist might look for to assess the effectiveness of integrating positive feeling words.

1. When the exercise is completed successfully, the client will take a deep releasing breath like a sigh,

2. Clients whose faces looked pale before the exercise often have more colour after the exercise is completed,

3. There will be a visible relaxing of the face and body.

Clients' observations regarding their experience:

Clients will say they feel a warm sensation either connected to where the pain was or radiating through their bodies. As the emotional feeling word of pain was released in Jan's exercise, the warm feeling was in her neck and shoulders, although, sometimes it is in other parts of the body as well, e.g., the centre of the chest, or the legs or hands, etc.

The radiation of warmth and the release of tension will indicate to you, the therapist, that the therapy has been successful.

Ask your client if they feel lighter, ask them if they feel as though a burden has been lifted. The answer will be in the affirmative and clients will share their own thoughts on what they are experiencing. Generally, theirs is a positive response; they will say things look brighter. The light itself looks more brilliant, colours are clearer, the trees outside the window look more defined and the feeling of pain has subsided or gone. Often, clients say they feel less confused.

On the success of the exercise ask your client if the picture they were working with is still there? If the work has been completed successfully the answer will be 'no', do not allow your client to search for the picture; explain that the memory of e.g., the accident or incident is still there, but the picture connected to the shock of what happened has gone or is lighter. Whether the neck pain has gone or not, depends on how much more therapy and physical body work, (e.g., massage or physiotherapy) the client needs, and sometimes the picture is still there but very light, not as defined as it was before which means that more Therapy is required.

'TRAUMA THERAPY' ALLOWS PRIVACY FOR CLIENTS.

In the early 1990s when I first started to realise how efficient and safe 'Trauma Therapy' was, a middle-aged man came to see me. He came because his partner had been to see me previously and told him about this 'wonderful' therapy. She told him that he did not need to tell his whole story, and when he came to see me, I respected his wish not to tell me the full details of what happened to him.

The shortened version of his story is that he did something wrong when he was a young man and had done some jail time. However, twenty years later, he said he could not let go of the original picture from his mind's eye and no matter what he did, mindfulness meditation, yoga etc., the continual dialogue that went on and on in his head never stopped, and he felt as if he was going crazy.

Using 'Trauma Therapy' revealed that his emotional feeling words were fear, hate, and anger.

I did not hear from him for quite a few months and then randomly I saw him on the street walking towards me. I asked him how he was going, he answered and said that slowly and surely life was becoming more normal. He said he was very relieved that the chatter in his mind was not as bad as it had been before he came to see me, adding that, generally, his life was more peaceful. A successful session, as far as it went, and a very unusual one, most clients do share their stories, willingly and want to come back for me to check on how they are going.

ADVANCED WORK FOR THERAPISTS

Belief Systems!

If, when questioned about his/her name a client says they are not getting an answer, it could be because:

1. the inner name they are being given is not the same as their own, or,

2. there is no answer, or,

3. maybe they use a nickname in ordinary everyday life. Then, because their answers do not follow the normal question and answer format of 'Trauma Therapy', more information is needed before the client and therapist can continue.

Always remember, your client has the answer. It is their agenda you are working with, not yours. Ask simple, closed questions that elicit 'yes' or 'no' answers to get the best results. Sometimes, at this point, the therapist should let go of the whole process if resistance is strong and ongoing.

Therapists who continue at this point need to establish that there is a picture and a recognisable first or nickname to work with before an emotional feeling word can be identified and released.

Emotional feeling words can be many and varied, such as — hate, anger, protection, shock, and they can also be real names such as Mary or John.

Hate, anger, protection, and shock are easy words to understand. However, words that are real ... names can also be emotional feeling words, real names such as Mary and John.

How they are to be dealt with will only be revealed during a session. These names may be connected in some way to the person in therapy, but they could also be thought of as religious names and might, therefore, indicate possession by some other energy, or person. This is not a possession in the religious, spiritual or ghostly sense, they are just words, emotional feeling words which should be named and released in the same way as any other emotional feeling word. The 'Trauma Therapy' format is followed in the same way in every session.

No matter what the emotional feeling word is, it is dealt with in the same way so that release and reconnection can come about.

If your client questions this information, explain to them that hearing a real name is unusual, that it does not happen to everyone and that it is still an emotional feeling word that needs to be identified and released in the normal way. Reassure your client that this has happened before and tell them they are safe and that they can trust the process.

ADVANCED THERAPY

The only time a therapist might decide to address this session differently is when a client has a different belief system. Having a different belief system might require using a different dialogue.

For example, if another name is recognised by a woman client and the name is Mary, the client might have a belief system that says, Mary the Mother of Jesus will protect her, or, it could mean that her Aunty Mary, who died, is there to help and protect her.

All names are emotional feeling words and occasionally a short discussion is needed to clarify the situation so that the wording of the therapy can be changed to match each different situation.

Belief systems impact clients because of their cultural or religious overtones; therefore, therapists are encouraged to acknowledge different cultures and belief systems. For instance, many people believe in and have different theories and ideas about good and evil and heaven and hell. When talking about heaven and hell, some clients will think of heaven as being above their heads, while hell is below their feet, others will think heaven and hell is all around them.

Understanding and respecting different belief systems means that the language of 'Trauma Therapy' can be adjusted to any culture or religion worldwide, e.g., Jewish, Roman Catholic, Buddhism, Muslim, or Spanish, Japanese, French, Chinese, Hindi, etc.

I write this here because of the research I have done into the global effect of shock and trauma. Worldwide diagnosing, treating and the healing of trauma and PTSD is challenging us all because — **shock does not discriminate, we are all susceptible!**

CHANGING THE DIALOGUE ENABLES THE THERAPIST TO ACKNOWLEDGE THE CLIENT'S BELIEF SYSTEMS, MEANING THAT 'TRAUMA THERAPY' CAN BE USED FOR ANYONE, ANYWHERE IN THE WORLD, IN ANY CULTURE, IN ANY LANGUAGE.

Emotional feeling words such as Mary and John are exactly that, emotional feeling words just like any other words such as protection, or control, hate or anger. The only difference is that we change the dialogue slightly to get the results we want.

In conversation, at the end of the session, some clients will tell quite interesting stories about protection. Some say they have never felt protected. Others say they believe they have always been protected, that, e.g., Mary, the Mother of Jesus, would always be there to protect them. Some will say, I feel as though Aunty Mary is still with me and will protect me. And, some will say my brother John died when I was young, but I have always believed that he is looking after me. Everyone's belief system is different, what is right for one person may not be right for another. Using 'Trauma Therapy' correctly will identify whether it is necessary to make alterations to the dialogue to be effective.

If a client releases an emotional feeling word such as Mary or John they feel the usual flow of warmth somewhere in their bodies, afterward they feel entirely different, and they often say, much safer, safer than at any time since childhood or at least since the time of an original shock.

Therapists may doubt this phenomenon. However, I include these examples here because as therapists see more clients they will become more adept at using 'Trauma Therapy'. As practitioners, therapists will come across increasingly more challenging sessions, because, it seems to me that there is a Universal Law that says the higher the achievement the more we are challenged. Therefore they will find themselves having to lateral think about how to adjust to different and, therefore, more challenging sessions.

CLIENTS FEEL VERY RELIEVED WHEN ANY INTERFERING EMOTIONAL FEELING WORD IS NAMED AND DEALT WITH WHETHER IT IS A PERSON'S NAME OR NOT; POSITIVE OR NEGATIVE, RECOGNISED OR UNRECOGNISED.

The only other explanation I can give therapists and clients alike to help them understand this phenomena is to again remind them that shock affects everyone in the same way — momentarily they separate from themselves, the mind at the same time takes a picture of the event and internalises an emotional feeling word.

At the instant of separation clients internalise whatever feeling word their belief system recognises, e.g., protection, or a belief that someone, e.g., Mary or John will help them, or be with them in times of stress. It is the original separation/disconnection plus the internalised emotional feeling word that causes people to feel different. Different from the person they were before they experienced the shock and were traumatised.

After the emotional feeling word is identified, integrated or released, clients say they feel much better, they say they feel 'connected,' 'together' or 'attached' again.

The feeling word is the key. 'Trauma Therapy' proves over and over again that the *emotional feeling word* is the key to the success of healing trauma.

Certain words such as trauma, shock and traumatised are not easily recognised by the general public, mainly because they do not know the meaning of the words. I would suggest that therapists use every- day ordinary words if they need to help a client who is at a loss for words.

Many people do not know that they have suffered a shock and are traumatised.

When using 'Trauma Therapy' to help with treating physical problems, it is a good idea to recognise 'physical' emotional feeling words, even if sometimes they do not sound like emotional feeling words, for example, walk, move, amble, crawl, stand, stand up, strength and strong, as integration words.

THE SUBCONSCIOUS TAKES EVERYTHING LITERALLY. THEREFORE, USING SIMPLE DESCRIPTIVE WORDS SUCH AS — INTEGRATE, COME, COMBINE WITH ME, STOP AND START ARE AS IMPORTANT AS THE NAMED 'EMOTIONAL FEELING WORD' WHEN SEEKING TO GET POSITIVE RESULTS FROM A SESSION.

'Trauma Therapy' is safe! It is another 'tool' to be added to the repertoire of the therapist. If you, the reader, decides that this therapy is for you, I wish you well and believe, that if you include the stress and anxiety management program that I have written about in my other book in your healing program, you will have a greater understanding of the process of healing.

SHORT SUMMARY

When the nervous system is affected by shock, it causes the body and mind to automatically go into survival mode. Some shocks are over quickly. Others, however, leave people chronically traumatised suffering PTSD for years.

AN EASY WAY TO RECOGNISE IF A PERSON IS TRAUMATISED IS TO ASK THEM IF THEY HAVE A PICTURE IN THEIR MIND'S EYE THAT THEY CANNOT LET GO OF.

If the answer is yes, then using the Principles of 'Trauma Therapy' may help them release the picture.

When doing the original work on myself I had no physical evidence of any other damage that I knew of, that is, until the next morning when the bruises in my neck became obvious after having released the emotional feeling word 'terrified' when using 'Trauma Therapy' on myself the night before. Deep down inside myself, however, I knew I still needed to do more therapy on the original unclear picture of the attack that was still in my mind's eye and eventually I released the attached emotional feeling word — fear.

When I acknowledged and released my emotional feeling word — fear, I realised that all my life I had lived in fear. Fear of everything and everyone! Fear and adrenaline had always controlled me.

I had subtly withdrawn, lived under and held my PTSD umbrella close to me for decades.

In the early years of my life, my father's generational PTSD affected us all. In later years, my personal PTSD caused me to hold my own umbrella even closer. Eventually I recognised that I needed to hold the last very unclear picture, of my personal attack, the one I could still see in my mind's eye, recognise the attached emotional feeling word, which was 'fear', and let it go. After I released my emotional feeling word, fear, I felt light and free.

It really was a wonderful feeling, a very pleasant physical experience when I finally released my fear. All the muscles in the lower part of my neck, at the back, around my shoulders started relaxing. I felt radiating warmth in the centre of my chest and in my neck.

Physically, after the attack in 1970, I was unable to bend my head back and look up at the sky without supporting my head in my hands. Now I can! Also, now the skin over the affected area at the base of my skull, at the back of my neck and across my shoulders is soft; before the release, it was very firm and painful to touch. After the release, I felt released on all levels — mentally, physically and emotionally.

PTSD is thought of as being a long term, severe, life-threatening disorder, which in many cases, it is. However, there are also other cases when the hidden levels of stress, anxiety, and PTSD that a person is suffering from, if recognised, can be treated successfully using 'Trauma Therapy'.

This book is an introduction to treating PTSD. It is meant to be both a teaching aid and a practical tool to help those who are interested in understanding and healing the after- effect of shock called trauma.

Ask yourself: 'is there a picture in my mind's eye of a shock I've had that will not go away?'

If there is a picture there, then, think about using 'Trauma Therapy' to release the emotional feeling word that is attached to that picture and release it.

'Trauma Therapy' is an easy to understand therapy which we can use to help in the healing of trauma. The five step program allows us to follow what is happening throughout the session. It helps us feel as though we have some control over what is going on and the most important thing for us is that we feel safe.

Some years ago, I ran a one-day workshop for a diverse group of about thirty people.

I thought the participants would be average everyday people who just wanted to know how to stop feeling stressed and anxious and at the same time learn something about diagnosing and treating trauma.

We were all settled and about to start when another group of about ten people walked into the room asking if they could join in, saying they had just read about the workshop.

The organisation itself was a high-profile organisation in a capital city, and the people who walked in were their trained counsellors, therapists, and Ph.Ds.

I felt overwhelmed for a few seconds at the thought of teaching this highly educated, much larger group. But all went well; they were an easy and cooperative group to work with.

Teaching them how to deal with stress and anxiety was pleasantly easy. Everyone took part and enjoyed themselves appreciating the practical success of learning how to breathe correctly.

To give the participants practice in how to use 'Trauma Therapy', I divided them into smaller groups of three, one person to observe and two to work with each other, one as the client and one as the therapist.

Everything went smoothly throughout the afternoon, and I can remember breathing a sigh of relief as I realised that both professionals and non-professionals are equally as receptive as one another to receiving this new information.

As I was standing there thinking the above thoughts, for a moment there was dead silence throughout the room as sometimes happens at the end of a successfully run workshop. Into this silence a voice to my right was heard saying, 'we are all doing it wrong', (counselling that is). One of the PhDs had summed up in a few words why 'Trauma Therapy' was so successful, it is able to do in a few minutes what had taken hours to do in the past and that is, take the stress out of counselling by shortening the time needed to get results. How rewarding for me was it to hear those few words, and I felt even more joyful when I heard others clapping in agreement.

This day's workshop had proved to me that 'Trauma Therapy' was both complete within itself and a program that medical, non-medical clinicians and the general public could master.

PART III
Trauma Therapy (shortened version)

Following is an example of how to understand and use the format of the simplest form of 'Trauma Therapy.'

'TRAUMA THERAPY' (shortened version)

Step 1. **Ask** your client if they, '*have a picture* in their mind's eye of a previous incident which was a shock'. If the answer is, '**yes**', say to them focus on the picture. Then say to your client, the picture is yours no matter who or what else is in the picture. (One of the key phrases from the client is: 'I can remember when!').

Step 2. Say to your client that you want them to identify with themselves in the picture by saying silently, (not aloud), to themselves, '*Is your name, e.g., Jan/ Peter?*' Always use your client's familiar name — this could be a nickname or a childhood name, or the name they are known by today. They will hear their own answer; the answer will be 'yes'.

Step 3. Ask your client to quietly say to their inner self, '*What are you feeling?*' They will hear the answer in their mind. It will be an emotional 'feeling' word, e.g., fear, hurt, pain, etc. Ask your client to tell you what their feeling word is. They will answer with an emotional feeling word, e.g., '**fear**'.

Step 4. Then ask your client to say to him/herself: '*Do you want to let the feeling of fear go?*' Usually, the answer the client hears is, '**Yes**'.

Step 5. Using the feeling word they have just given you, ask them to say to their inner self, '*Let the feeling of, e.g., fear go, come towards me, integrate with me and come through to where I am now.* **Stop feeling fear and start feeling safe.**' Usually, the client releases a big sigh of relief as the feeling of fear dissipates and they reconnect with their disconnected self.

To clarify that the work is complete I then ask my client if the picture has gone. Then I ask if they have a warm feeling somewhere? They will answer that the picture has gone, and they feel warm, e.g., in the solar plexus, (stomach), or the heart centre. Clients say they feel relieved as if a burden has been lifted from them, they feel lighter, more relaxed and calmer and they usually look happier and more relaxed.

PART IV: UPDATE — 2017
Trauma Free, Your Five Steps to Freedom.

If you read the introduction to this book — *Trauma Free, Your Five Steps to Freedom* - about the various names Post Traumatic Stress Disorder, (PTSD), has been known by over the years, you would have noticed that I added a new name to the list — **Post Emotional Shock/Trauma, (PEST)**, the reason for this update is because I had, in early 2020, an amazing breakthrough, concerning my understanding of the basic difference between mental, (PTSD), and emotional, (PEST), illness.

The following pages summarize the shift in thinking I had regarding the diagnosis and treatment of mental and emotional illness. Once the differences became clear to me, it was easy to separate the diagnosis and treatment of emotional illness from mental illness. Separation and this new light-bulb moment of shocked understanding helped me get improved results from the work I was already doing.

PART V:
An Overview and Conclusion 2020

Trauma Free, Your Five Steps to Freedom has taken me about twenty-five years to write and because of the circumstances of my life it has been written from my point of view only. In some parts it describes in detail my life of suffering from what was thought to have been a conventional mental health illness relating to trauma called Post Traumatic Stress Disorder, PTSD. I did not at any time really believe that I was mental and during those long years I asked myself many questions about what was wrong with me and have, with clarity come to a new conclusion concerning what was really wrong with me.

As a result of my research I have come to the conclusion that my problems were emotional in origin, rather than mental in origin, and I have coined a new phrase and acronym to describe the change — **Post Emotional Shock/Trauma, PEST.**

This new phrase and acronym clearly shows the difference between mental and emotional illnesses. By association, PTSD is considered to be a mental disorder, however, by including the word emotional in the new phrase and acronym it is easy to see that trauma is an emotional disorder rather than a mental disorder.

The following is an overview of some of the difficulties I had to overcome within my own thinking before I could arrive at that conclusion.

Early on, I realised that I was not mental. Knowing I thought differently from others who thought I was mental, isolated me and made me more determined than ever to find out what was wrong with me. Gradually, as the years went by, I succeeded in finding an answer.

Over decades, acceptance of who I was and am today became the first lesson I needed to learn. The second lesson was to know that it was okay for me to be different, to stay on the path I was on and continue developing both the storyline of my book, *Trauma Free, Your Five Steps to Freedom* and 'Trauma Therapy', the therapy that eventually saved, and changed my life.

Using the five steps of 'Trauma Therapy', I have healed myself and in doing so have given myself absolute proof that there is a big difference between PTSD — mental illness, and PEST emotional illness. Over the years I had to train myself to use the principles of 'Trauma Therapy' in a disciplined way to get the results I wanted, i.e. to be healthy. I did eventually train myself to remember to work on myself and successfully and repeatedly proved to myself that my problems were 'emotional' in origin rather than 'mental' in origin.

To separate PTSD a mental illness from an emotional illness, I have added a new phrase and acronym to the list of trauma disorder phrases and acronyms –**PEST, Post Emotional Shock/Trauma**. PEST accurately describes what was wrong with me. I had an emotionally-based illness which caused me to be traumatised. I was traumatised after suffering many <u>emotional shocks</u> — Post (meaning after), an Emotional Shock, (comes) Trauma.

In the 1990s when I first heard about medically diagnosed PTSD, a mental illness I felt devastated, because deep down I knew that other people, family mainly, thought there was something mentally wrong with me.

I was utterly amazed to think that I might have PTSD a 'mental' disorder. I already knew because of the work I was doing developing 'Trauma Therapy' that I did not have a mental disorder of any kind. I knew I had an 'emotional' disorder! I knew I did not have a mental illness because I was getting really good results using 'Trauma Therapy' to heal myself from some of the shocks and trauma I had suffered over the years.

'Trauma Therapy' worked! How did I know? I knew because I was feeling better than I had done for years, I could think more clearly, my energy levels were coming up and I was feeling less depressed and lonely. I knew, by identifying and releasing the *emotional feeling words* connected to the many *pictures* stored in my subconscious when using 'Trauma Therapy' that I was gradually finding my answers because healing followed.

One of the hardest things to master, when healing oneself, is the discipline of using and believing in the work one is doing.

I knew that I needed to be disciplined myself regarding remembering to use 'Trauma Therapy'. Whenever I found life hard-going, I did the work and I should like to add here that every time I used 'Trauma Therapy' successfully, I was reminded that I did not have a mental disorder. This can be a slow way to heal but heal me it did causing me to eventually become 'trauma-free'.

My main concern, however, had always been why couldn't I connect with family members? As I thought about this I realised that they may have labelled me mental and an embarrassment to them years ago. I wondered if their collective point of view had labelled me mental and that is why I could not connect with them.

As those thoughts went through my mind, I felt a shift in

me as understanding flooded my thinking. Up to that time I blamed myself for everything that was wrong but now I could see that it takes two to create relationships. One single person cannot make changes without the cooperation of others, and there was, I already knew, absolutely no cooperation between me and other family members in my family regarding letting our unhappy past go.

I knew without a doubt that I did not carry the stigma, or label, of 'mental illness' and PTSD. What a relief I thought. What a feeling that sense of relief gave me as it surged through me when I realised I was only suffering from Post Emotional Shock/Trauma, (PEST), an emotional disorder. At last, I thought, I can relax and let go of some of my feelings of guilt and shame about my family. I knew at last, I could let go because I knew I was relatively normal.

Post Emotional Shock/Trauma — PEST is not a mental illness as Post Traumatic Stress Disorder — PTSD is! In my opinion there are no similarities whatsoever.

PTSD implies because it is a diagnosed psychiatric disorder, that it is a mental problem. Psychiatrists diagnose and treat mental illness, whereas, 'Trauma Therapy' is concerned with issues that are emotional in origin only.

As I tested my theories it became glaringly obvious to me that the gap between diagnosing and treating PTSD and PEST was enormous. It appeared to me that there were no areas of crossover or similarity between diagnosing and treating mental and emotional illness.

What a revelation; I was blown away with the enormity of my discovery!

PEST is a person's normal automatic emotional response to shock. As the nervous system goes into shock, the body and mind spontaneously respond by altering the physical body's normal breathing pattern. The mind takes a picture of what the eyes see at the time of the incident, internalises an emotional feeling word, and trauma follows. PEST is the physical body's mental, physical and emotional response to emotional shock. First there is shock and then there is trauma!

For me being attacked and strangled and left for dead on my bedroom floor and then losing my baby, sight unseen straight down the toilet the next morning were huge shocks. I was severely traumatised for decades by these events, but having been discharged from a mental hospital with a clean bill of health after voluntarily admitting myself there, I knew two things as I travelled through life; first, that I wasn't mental and, second, I was absolutely certain that 'Trauma Therapy' would eventually heal me.

Trauma is on a continuum. At one end of the scale, trauma is severe at the other end it is less severe, and it is important to remember here that healing may be gradual because we internalise many shocks over a lifetime. Know that each shock has a different level of impact. Therefore, the levels of trauma after each shock vary. To assess the impact of shock and the resulting trauma, it is important to follow carefully the guidelines of the system of diagnosis and treatment set down in 'Trauma Therapy'. 'Trauma Therapy' proves itself. If there is no picture in the mind's eye and there is no emotional word to work with then there is no use for the 'five steps' of 'Trauma Therapy'. If responses to the questions asked in 'Trauma Therapy' are unsatisfactory, another form of therapy should be chosen.

It was so simple and so easy. All I had to do to heal myself was remember to continue to use 'Trauma Therapy', release the 'emotional feeling words' connected to the 'pictures' in my mind's eye and give my mind and body time to heal.

For years I lived with the fear of the stigma of being labelled 'mental'. This fear slowed my progress considerably because I felt as though I should prove to everyone that I was normal. However, many minds around me were already set in stone and I could not change them. It took me years to realise that I could not force anyone to change, years to realise that the only person I could change was me. A lonely journey but acceptance is a great gift. If we can accept, learn and grow from any journey, we become much more acceptable people, even if it is only to ourselves. Gradually the therapy and the knowledge that I was not mental released me, and much of my fear went with it.

With knowledge came happiness! All I wanted to do was jump up and down and share my happiness and information with others; I wanted to shout to the world that I was normal, not mental. I wanted them to know that I was NOT MENTAL. Sadly, to this day I have little contact with family members, and recently when I asked one estranged member if he wanted to read this book, he said, 'I don't care what you do, I don't care,' so things haven't changed.

Ask yourself, 'do you have a picture in your mind's eye that *you* can release?' 'Trauma Therapy' is an easy, simple system to understand and use and Post Emotional Shock/Trauma, (PEST) is easy to diagnose and treat.

Ask yourself are you suffering PTSD — Post-Traumatic Stress Disorder, a mental disorder, or PEST — Post Emotional Shock/Trauma, an emotional disorder? Test yourself by asking yourself the relevant questions and listen to your answers as you follow the format of 'Trauma Therapy'.

As I thought about the difference between the two disorders most of my feelings of guilt and shame left me. Also, as this shift happened I had a light bulb moment and thought to myself, I wonder if this is one of the reasons why people don't go and ask for help when they know there is something wrong,

I wondered if, like me, they feared being labelled 'mental'? I had seen it happen to others! If we are labelled 'mental,' that label follows us as a stigma for the rest of our lives and generationally our children and grandchildren are also labelled.

I pondered this dilemma for a few years wondering if I could do anything about it. That is why, in my retirement years, very much against the wishes of my estranged family who know that I have self-published this book, I have decided to finish it and find a publisher. Then, hopefully take the information further by publishing it in other languages and circulating it worldwide so that others can help themselves if they choose to. I do not like the label 'mental'. I do not want to be labelled as such myself, and I imagine others feel the same way.

I don't know much about Post-Traumatic-Stress Disorder as a mental illness; I did know, however, that there was still more to come after I wrote about stress and anxiety in my other published book. Realising that I was severely emotionally traumatised by what I went through I wanted more answers. I wanted to know how I could fully get my life back on track.

Personally, I feel much better about myself owning the truth that I was 'emotionally' ill, PEST, rather than 'mentally' ill, PTSD, and humbly today, in my eightieth year, I think I am living proof of the truth of the above statement, because, in allowing for my age, I know I am doing quite well.

I do here add, however, that I sometimes still question my diagnosis of myself and need my friends to reassure me that my problems were and are emotional in origin, not mental. I reassure myself by thinking how could I have healed myself, survived so well the sometimes insurmountable problems that faced me and put the work needed into developing a new therapy, 'Trauma Therapy' if I was mentally ill. The answer to that is — I don't think I could have done it if I was mentally ill because, even though I knew there was something wrong, my mind proved time and time again that, thank goodness, it still had the capacity to think, reason and make decisions.

'Trauma Therapy' is a simple, easy to understand, practical therapy that has worked for me and it can work for you. Ask yourself, 'will it work for me?'. If the answer comes back 'yes,' find someone you can work with and go through the 'Therapy' together. Being labelled 'a PEST' is more acceptable than being labelled PTSD in this intellectual, mind-driven world we live in today.

The choice is yours. If you are uncertain about what to do always consult your healthcare person for advice.

I wish you every success

www.ingramcontent.com/pod-product-compliance
Lightning Source LLC
Chambersburg PA
CBHW021153080526
44588CB00008B/310